The Leiden Developmental Care Project:

Effects of developmental care on behavior and quality of life of very preterm infants and parental and staff experiences

Leiden University Press

Leiden University Press is an imprint of Amsterdam University Press

The Leiden Developmental Care Project described in this thesis was financially supported by: ZONMW (grant 2100.0072) and the Doelmatigheidsfonds LUMC.

Financial support for the publication of this thesis was provided by: Jurriaanse Stichting, Nycomed B.V. and Abbott B.V.

Cover illustration: István de Koning (Lina Geibreen)
Cover design: Randy Lemaire, Utrecht
Lay-out: István de Koning

isbn 978 90 8728 019 2
nur 870

The Leiden Developmental Care Project:

Effects of developmental care on behavior and quality of life of very preterm infants and parental and staff experiences.

PROEFSCHRIFT

ter verkrijging van
de graad van Doctor aan de Universiteit Leiden,
op gezag van de Rector Magnificus,
prof.mr. P.F. van der Heijden,
volgens besluit van het College voor Promoties
te verdedigen op dinsdag 17 april 2007
klokke 15:00 uur

door

Sylvia Maria van der Pal

geboren te Leidschendam,
in 1980

Promotiecommissie

Promotores:	Prof. Dr. F.J. Walther
	Prof. Dr. J.M. Wit
Co-promotor:	Dr. J. Bruil
Referent:	Prof. Dr. S.P. Verloove-Vanhorick
Overige leden:	Prof. Dr. A.A. Kaptein
	Prof. Dr. I.A. Van Berckelaer-Onnes
	Prof. Dr. S. Maes

TABLE OF CONTENTS

CHAPTER 1

Introduction

Preterm birth: infants and their parents

Advances in neonatal caregiving have decreased the mortality of infants born very preterm [1,2]. When an infant is born preterm this also has a major long-lasting impact on both the family and the individual infant. Parents of preterm infants report more stress [3,4] and experience more maladaptation and need for support during the first year after delivery [5] than parents of infants born at term. Furthermore, mothers of high-risk preterm infants have reported that they experience symptoms of post-traumatic stress [6].

Very preterm infants have lower health-related quality of life (HRQoL) compared to children born at term [7-10], as reported by their parents, especially regarding stomach, lungs and eating problems [9]. Health-related quality of life is defined as the functioning of the child on four dimensions (physical functioning, social functioning, cognitive functioning and emotional functioning), weighted by the emotional evaluation of the problems [11,12]. Preterm infants also show more problem behavior compared to infants born at term. A meta-analysis [13] found more externalizing and internalizing problem behavior in preterm infants in 13 out of 16 studies (81%) and more Attention Deficit and Hyperactivity Disorder (ADHD) symptom behavior in 10 out of 15 studies (67%).

Parental stress and infant behavior problems are interrelated in which increased maternal stress and depression at 4 months and parents' post traumatic stress reactions were correlated with increased problem behavior at 36 months [14] and increased risk of the child developing sleeping and eating problems [15].

The NIDCAP intervention

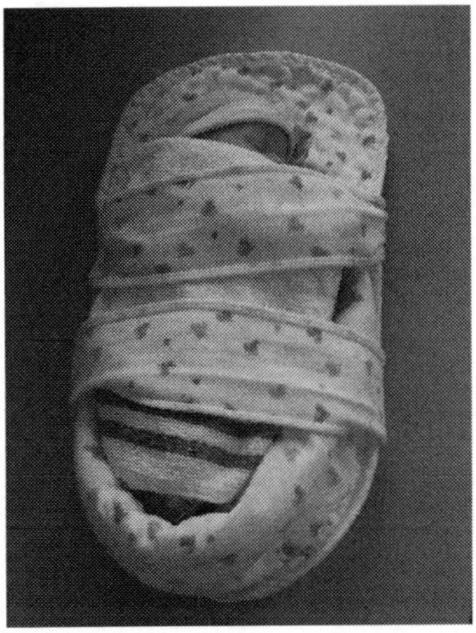

Because of the advances in neonatal caregiving and the decrease in the mortality of infants born preterm [1,2], focus in neonatal caregiving has shifted to a more individualized and family-centered approach. In this context the Newborn Individualized Developmental Care and Assessment Program (NIDCAP) [16], introduced by dr. Heidelise Als in the 1980's, seems very promising. This program is based on the Synactive Theory of Development [17] where the infant's behavior is observed along four channels of communication: the autonomic system (skin color, respiration etc.), the motor system (posture, tone and movements), the state organization system (type and range of states available to the infant from asleep to aroused and state transition) and the attention and interaction system (the infant's ability to come to an alert, attentive state and to utilize this state to handle stimuli from the environment). The infant's efforts at self-regulation and interaction are observed through approach and avoidance behaviors [17,18]. The infant's behavior is observed before, during and after caregiving by a NIDCAP trained developmental specialist. A narrative of the observation is written with recommendations to modify the infant's environment and caregiving, based on the infant's individual behavior. Examples of recommendations are: time-outs during caregiving when the infant becomes stressed, giving the infant something to hold on to or to suck on (whatever comforts the infant most) and placing the caregiver's hands around the infant's body to support flexed position and to provide comforting boundaries (containing). Furthermore, parents are guided in observing and responding to the infant's behavioral cues during caregiving and kangaroo care is encouraged (placing the infant on the parent's chest to support bonding and provide the infant with familiar odours, sounds and warmth). The observations and recommendations are discussed with parents and other caregivers and parents are stimulated to become more actively involved in the caregiving process [16,19].

The results of NIDCAP intervention studies in the United States and Sweden revealed improved infant outcomes, such as improved short term medical outcomes (fewer ventilation days, shorter duration of parenteral feeding and lower incidence of necrotizing enterocolitis) [20-22], better behavioral performance as measured with the Assessment of Preterm Behavior (APIB) [20,21,23-25], improved cognitive developmental outcome [18,21,23,26], lower hospital charges [26], improved brain function and altered brain structure [23] and a positive impact on behavior [27]. In addition, less parental stress was reported [20]. However, a recent review regarding Developmental Care [28] concluded that although overall limited benefits and no major harmful effects were found, the significant effects were mainly based on studies with small sample sizes and that several of these findings were not supported in other settings.

Basic Developmental Care

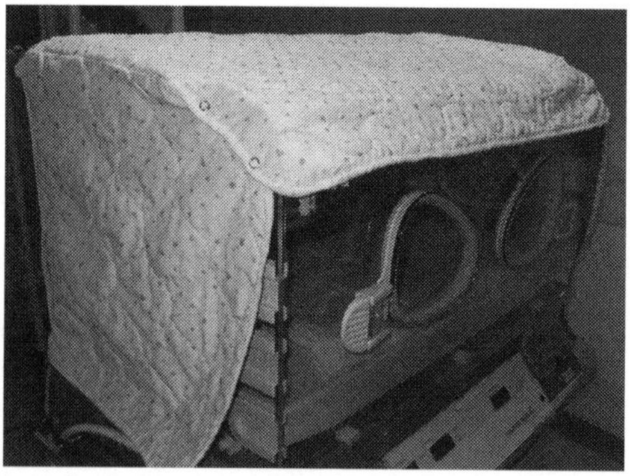

The NIDCAP observations have resulted in basic recommendations for the Neonatal Intensive Care Unit (NICU) such as the use of standardized nests (to support the children's posture) and standardized incubator covers (to decrease the light level in the incubator). The guidance by a NIDCAP trained developmental specialist, the NIDCAP training and the individual observations are (labor) intensive and costly to implement. In this context the implementation of the basic recommendations of Developmental Care can be seen as a first step before deciding to officially train staff members. Previous research has only focused on the implementation of the complete NIDCAP observations. A comparison of the basic elements of Developmental Care with the complete and more intensive NIDCAP intervention would provide information about the additional value of the individualized aspects of the NIDCAP observations and guidance by a NIDCAP trained developmental specialist.

Implementation of NIDCAP in a Dutch setting

The implementation of NIDCAP in a NICU is very intensive and requires changes in the NICU environment and care as well as changes in medical and nursing staff's attitudes. Als and Gilkerson [19] stated that because NIDCAP is relationship-based, system-orientated, process-guided and not procedure-based, it can be difficult to implement NIDCAP in an acute care environment like the NICU, which focuses on medical protocols and caregiving routines [19].

A study of NIDCAP in a Swedish setting examined staff experiences and opinions regarding the implementation of NIDCAP. This study concluded that NIDCAP was well-received by nursing staff, neonatologists and parents [29,30]. Staff indicated improvements with regards to their ability to assess the infant, the infant's well-being and the opportunities for, and quality of, parental attachment. Because the implementation phase can influence the acceptance of NIDCAP in the unit it is important to monitor and evaluate NIDCAP implementation. The evaluation of NIDCAP implementation can result in recommendations for future implementation in different settings.

Study design

The study described in this thesis consists of two consecutive randomized controlled trails (RCT) evaluating the effects of NIDCAP in two stages (basic and complete Developmental Care) in a Dutch Neonatal Center at two locations (Leiden and The Hague). In addition, the nursing and (para)medical staff's experience with NIDCAP and attitudes at both locations were evaluated. The Neonatal Center encompasses 8 Intensive Care beds and 8 High Care beds in the level III unit in the Leiden University Medical Center (LUMC) and 4 Intensive Care beds and 9 High Care beds in the level III unit in the Juliana Children's Hospital in The Hague. Usually, infants admitted to the LUMC remain there until they are stable and are transferred to a medium care unit in a regional hospital, where they remain until they are discharged to go home. Infants admitted to the Juliana Children's Hospital usually remain in the unit until they are discharged to go home.

During the first RCT (inclusion period: April 2000 – March 2002) we evaluated the effect of the basic elements of Developmental Care (DC). The intervention was based on the reduction of light and sound through the use of standardized incubator covers and the support of motor development and physiological stability by positioning the infant in ways that encourage flexion and containment through the use of standardized nests. The control group received standard care without incubator covers or forms of nesting.

During the second RCT (inclusion period: July 2002- August 2004) we evaluated the additional effect of individual care plans and guidance through the use of the NIDCAP behavioral and observation tool [16,19]. The intervention in the second trial consisted of NIDCAP observations of the infant before, during and after caregiving [16] every 7 to 10 days by a NIDCAP-trained developmental specialist. The trained developmental specialist wrote reports and discussed recommendations with parents and other caregivers and supported them in giving care to the infant. The first observation was done within 48 hours after birth. The control group in the second trial received the basic elements of DC as described in the first trial.

The parents were given questionnaires measuring parental stress, confidence and perceived nurse support after 1 week of their infant's birth. Parents also received a set of questionnaires, measuring parental stress, the child's health-related quality of life and child behavior at the follow-up appointments with the neonatologist at 1 and 2 years of their child's corrected age (age corrected for gestational age at birth, thus time interval from term date). During the second RCT an additional questionnaire measuring infant temperament was send to the home addresses of parents at 9 months of corrected age. A summary of the questionnaires and outcome measures described in this thesis is shown in Table 1.

The NIDCAP was implemented in the course of the two RCT's. After the two RCT's (2 years implementation of basic DC and 2 years implementation of NIDCAP), a questionnaire was given to the nursing and (para)medical personnel in both hospitals to evaluate their opinions regarding the implementation of NIDCAP.

We developed this study design to explore the effects of two forms of developmental care (basic DC and the NIDCAP observations and guidance) on parental stress and infant behavior and health-related quality of life. We furthermore wanted to report the parents' and nursing and (para)medical staff's experiences with NIDCAP. We expected the basic elements of developmental care to positively affect parental stress and infant behavior and health-related quality of life. Furthermore we expected the more individualized NIDCAP intervention to further increase the positive effect of the basic elements of developmental care, especially on parental stress, confidence and perceived nurse support and the infant's self-regulatory behavior.

	Questionnaire	Measuring	N RCT 1*	N RCT 2*	Ch.
After 1 week admission	Parental Stressor Scale - NICU	Parental stress	133	150	2
	Nurse Parent Support Tool	Nurse support	133	150	2
	Mothers and Baby Scale - 2 scales	Parental confidence	133	150	2
9 months corr. age	Infant Behavior Questionnaire - Revised	Infant temperament	Not given	134	5
1 year corr. age	TNO-AZL Preschool Quality of Life	Health related quality of life	136	128	3
	Infant-Toddler Social & Emotional Assessment	Infant behavior	139	128	4/5
	NOSIK, Nijmegen Parental Stress Index - short	Parental stress	139	128	4/5
2 years corr. age	Child Behavior Checklist 2-3 yrs	Infant problem behavior	133		4
	NOSI, Nijmegen Parental Stress Index	Parental stress	133		4
After both RCT's	Questionnaire NIDCAP Implementation	Staff attitudes (N=124)			6

Table 1. Questionnaires given during both RCT's

* Number of infants whose parents completed the questionnaire.

RCT 1: standard care - basic elements of Developmental Care, inclusion period: April 2000 – March 2002, 192 infants included.

RCT 2: basic elements of Developmental Care – NIDCAP (Newborn Individualized Developmental Care and Assessment Program), inclusion period: July 2002- August 2004, 168 infants included.

Outline of the thesis

The objective of this thesis was to measure the effect of the basic elements of developmental care and the complete NIDCAP on several parent and infant outcomes during admission and at 1 and 2 years of age. This thesis furthermore aims to report staff's attitudes after NIDCAP implementation in a Dutch NICU.

Chapter 2 describes the effect of the basic elements of developmental care (the use of standardized nests and covers) and the more individualized NIDCAP intervention on parental stress, confidence and perceived nurse support while the child is admitted to the neonatal intensive care unit.

Chapter 3 reports on the effect of both the basic developmental care and the NIDCAP intervention on the infant's health-related quality of life at 1 year of corrected age.

Chapter 4 describes the effect of the basic elements of developmental care, compared to standard care, on parental stress and child behavior at 1 and 2 years of corrected age.

Chapter 5 reports on the effect of the complete NIDCAP intervention, compared to basic developmental care, on parental stress, child behavior and temperament and parent's opinions during the infant's first year of life.

Chapter 6 evaluates the nursing and (para)medical staff's attitudes towards the implementation of NIDCAP after the two RCT's.

In conclusion, **Chapter 7** discusses the results of both trials and the implementation evaluation and discusses the conclusions and implications that can be derived from these outcomes.

References

1. Hansen,B.M. & Greisen,G. Is improved survival of very-low-birthweight infants in the 1980s and 1990s associated with increasing intellectual deficit in surviving children? *Dev. Med. Child Neurol.* **46**, 812-815 (2004).

2. Veen,S. *et al.* Impairments, disabilities, and handicaps of very preterm and very-low-birthweight infants at five years of age. The Collaborative Project on Preterm and Small for Gestational Age Infants (POPS) in The Netherlands. *Lancet* **338**, 33-36 (1991).

3. Lau,R. & Morse,C.A. Stress experiences of parents with premature infants in a special care nursery. *Stress and Health* **19**, 69-78 (2003).

4. Singer,L.T. *et al.* Maternal psychological distress and parenting stress after the birth of a very low-birth-weight infant. *JAMA* **281**, 799-805 (1999).

5. Rautava,P., Lehtonen,L., Helenius,H. & Sillanpaa,M. Effect of newborn hospitalization on family and child behavior: a 12-year follow-up study. *Pediatrics* **111**, 277-283 (2003).

6. Holditch-Davis,D., Bartlett,T.R., Blickman,A.L. & Miles,M.S. Posttraumatic stress symptoms in mothers of premature infants. *J. Obstet. Gynecol. Neonatal Nurs.* **32**, 161-171 (2003).

7. Klassen,A.F. *et al.* Health status and health-related quality of life in a population-based sample of neonatal intensive care unit graduates. *Pediatrics* **113**, 594-600 (2004).

8. Saigal,S. *et al.* Comparison of the health-related quality of life of extremely low birth weight children and a reference group of children at age eight years. *J. Pediatr.* **125**, 418-425 (1994).

9. Stoelhorst,G.M. Development, Quality of Life and Behavior at 2 Years of Age in Very Preterm Infants. Doctoral dissertation. Leiden University Medical Centre, Leiden (2003).

10. Theunissen,N.C. *et al.* Quality of life in preschool children born preterm. *Dev. Med. Child Neurol.* **43**, 460-465 (2001).

11. Vogels,T. *et al.* Measuring health-related quality of life in children: the development of the TACQOL parent form. *Qual. Life Res.* **7**, 457-465 (1998).

12. Verrips,E.G. *et al.* Measuring health-related quality of life in a child population. *Eur. J. Public Health* **9**, 188-193 (1999).

13. Bhutta,A.T., Cleves,M.A., Casey,P.H., Cradock,M.M. & Anand,K.J. Cognitive and behavioral outcomes of school-aged children who were born preterm: a meta-analysis. *JAMA* **288**, 728-737 (2002).

14. Miceli,P.J. *et al.* Brief report: birth status, medical complications, and social environment: individual differences in development of preterm, very low birth weight infants. *J. Pediatr. Psychol.* **25**, 353-358 (2000).

15. Pierrehumbert,B., Nicole,A., Muller-Nix,C., Forcada-Guex,M. & Ansermet,F. Parental post-traumatic reactions after premature birth: implications for sleeping and eating problems in the infant. *Arch. Dis. Child Fetal Neonatal Ed* **88**, F400-F404 (2003).

16. Als,H. Developmental Interventions in the Neonatal Intensive Care Nursery. Goldson,E. (ed.), pp. 18-85 (Oxford University Press, New York,1999).

17. Als,H. Towards a synactive theory of development: Promise for the assessment of infant individuality. *Infant Mental Health Journal* **3**, 229-243 (1982).

18. Kleberg,A., Westrup,B. & Stjernqvist,K. Developmental outcome, child behaviour and mother-child interaction at 3 years of age following Newborn Individualized Developmental Care and Intervention Program (NIDCAP) intervention. *Early Hum. Dev.* **60**, 123-135 (2000).

19. Als,H. & Gilkerson,L. The role of relationship-based developmentally supportive newborn intensive care in strengthening outcome of preterm infants. *Semin. Perinatol.* **21**, 178-189 (1997).

20. Als,H. *et al.* A three-center, randomized, controlled trial of individualized developmental care for very low birth weight preterm infants: medical, neurodevelopmental, parenting, and caregiving effects. *J. Dev. Behav. Pediatr.* **24**, 399-408 (2003).

21. Als,H. *et al.* Individualized developmental care for the very low-birth-weight preterm infant. Medical and neurofunctional effects. *JAMA* **272**, 853-858 (1994).

22. Westrup,B., Kleberg,A., von Eichwald,K., Stjernqvist,K. & Lagercrantz,H. A randomized, controlled trial to evaluate the effects of

the newborn individualized developmental care and assessment program in a Swedish setting. *Pediatrics* **105**, 66-72 (2000).

23. Als,H. *et al.* Early experience alters brain function and structure. *Pediatrics* **113**, 846-857 (2004).

24. Mouradian,L.E. & Als,H. The influence of neonatal intensive care unit caregiving practices on motor functioning of preterm infants. *Am. J. Occup. Ther.* **48**, 527-533 (1994).

25. Buehler,D.M., Als,H., Duffy,F.H., McAnulty,G.B. & Liederman,J. Effectiveness of individualized developmental care for low-risk preterm infants: behavioral and electrophysiologic evidence. *Pediatrics* **96**, 923-932 (1995).

26. Fleisher,B.E. *et al.* Individualized developmental care for very-low-birth-weight premature infants. *Clin. Pediatr. (Phila)* **34**, 523-529 (1995).

27. Westrup,B., Bohm,B., Lagercrantz,H. & Stjernqvist,K. Preschool outcome in children born very prematurely and cared for according to the Newborn Individualized Developmental Care and Assessment Program (NIDCAP). *Acta Paediatr.* **93**, 498-507 (2004).

28. Symington,A. & Pinelli,J. Developmental care for promoting development and preventing morbidity in preterm infants. *Cochrane. Database. Syst. Rev.* CD001814 (2006).

29. Westrup,B., Stjernqvist,K., Kleberg,A., Hellstrom-Westas,L. & Lagercrantz,H. Neonatal individualized care in practice: a Swedish experience. *Semin. Neonatol.* **7**, 447-457 (2002).

30. Westrup,B. *et al.* Evaluation of the Newborn Individualized Developmental Care and Assessment Program (NIDCAP) in a Swedish setting. *Prenatal and Neonatal Medicine* **2**, 366-375 (1997).

CHAPTER 2

Parental experiences during the admission of their very preterm infant after two Developmental Care interventions

LVIA M. VAN DER PAL
ELESTE M. MAGUIRE
SKIA LE CESSIE
N MAARTEN WIT
RANS J. WALTHER
ANET BRUIL

Abstract

Aim:

To explore the effect of two developmental care interventions on parental stress, confidence and perceived nursing support.

Methods:

Two consecutive randomized controlled trials comparing 1) standard care versus basic developmental care (standardized nests and incubator covers) (n=133) and 2) basic developmental care versus the Newborn Individualized Developmental Care and Assessment Program (NIDCAP) (n=150). Parents of infants born < 32 weeks gestational age completed questionnaires after the first week of admission.

Results:

No significant differences were found on parental stress, confidence or perceived nursing support. The difference in stress between mother and father tended to be less in the NIDCAP intervention group (p=.03).

Conclusion:

Both developmental care interventions had little effect on parental experiences during admission. As a result of increased paternal stress, the NIDCAP intervention tended to decrease the difference in stress levels of fathers and mothers, possibly because of the increased involvement of father during the NIDCAP intervention.

Introduction

The preterm birth of an infant is in most cases unexpected and overwhelming for parents. Parents of preterm infants report more stress [1,2] and experience more maladaptation and need for support during the first year after delivery [3] than parents of infants born at term. Mothers of high-risk preterm infants may furthermore experience symptoms of post-traumatic stress syndrome [4]. High parental distress, anxiety and posttraumatic stress is related to poorer parental and infant outcomes, such as: behavior, sleeping and eating problems, poorer developmental outcomes and less effective parental coping strategies [5-8].

Neonatal care has become more family-centered over the past years. The Newborn Individualized Developmental Care and Assessment Program (NIDCAP) [9] is an intervention based on the individuality of preterm infants and their families and was developed by Heidelise Als in the 1980's. This program is based on the Synactive Theory of Infant Development in which the infant's behavior is observed along four channels of communication: being the autonomic (color, respiration patterns, etc.), motor (posture, tone and movements), state organization (type and range of sleep and wake states available to the infant from asleep to aroused and state transition) and attention and interaction system (the infant's ability to come to an alert, attentive state and to utilize this state to handle stimuli from the environment). The infant's efforts at self-regulation and interaction are observed through approach and avoidance behaviors before, during and after caregiving by a trained developmental specialist. A narrative of the observation is written and discussed with parents and other caregivers as a guide for caregiving and for modifying the infant's environment [9].

The results of NIDCAP intervention studies in the United States and Sweden show positive infant outcomes [10-15]. The effect of NIDCAP on parental stress has been studied in Sweden [16] and in a three-center study in the USA [11]. In the three-center study, mothers of infants that had received NIDCAP indicated less parental stress and described their infant as being more independent when completing the Mother's View of the Child (MVC) compared to controls, two weeks after the expected date of confinement [11]. Recently, the effects of various developmental-care-based interventions were reviewed [17]. The interventions ranged from basic interventions, focused on positioning and modification of external stimuli, to more individualized developmental care interventions, such as the NIDCAP program. The authors concluded that overall limited benefits and no major harmful effects were found, but that the significant effects were mainly based on studies with small sample sizes and several of these findings were not supported in other settings.

The current study aims to explore the effect of a basic and less intensive form of developmental care (the use of standardized covers and nests) and the effect of the more intensive and individualized NIDCAP intervention (with individual behavior observations and guidance) on parental experiences during admission. Our hypothesis was that the basic elements of developmental care would reduce parental stress because infants may appear more comfortable to parents because of the incubator covers and nests. The more individualized NIDCAP intervention was thought to further reduce parental stress and increase parental confidence and the nurse support parents perceived. Previous studies have shown that mothers of preterm infants report more stress in comparison with fathers [18,19]. Our secondary hypothesis was that NIDCAP would decrease the difference in maternal and paternal stress levels because of the active inclusion of both parents in the caregiving process.

Methods

Developmental care interventions

Two consecutive randomized controlled trials (RCT's) at a tertiary NICU with two locations in the Netherlands were carried out to measure the effect of two Developmental Care interventions. The first randomized controlled trial (inclusion: April 2000 to May 2002) studied the effect of the basic elements of developmental care. The basic developmental care intervention consisted of the reduction of light and sound through the use of standardized incubator covers, which shielded the incubator on the top and three sides. Motor development and physiological stability were supported by using standardized nests and positioning aids to support a flexed position with boundaries. The control group received the standard care prior to the beginning of this research project, when no covers or nests were used.

The second randomized controlled trial (inclusion: July 2002 to August 2004) studied the additional effect of NIDCAP compared to the basic elements of developmental care. The intervention in the second trial consisted of NIDCAP observations of the infant's behavior before, during and after caregiving every 7 to 10 days by a NIDCAP-trained developmental specialist [9]. A psychologist and 5 nurses were trained to use the NIDCAP observational tool [9]. These trained developmental specialists wrote behavioral reports and discussed individualized recommendations with parents and other caregivers and supported them in giving care to the infant. The first observation was done within 48 hours after birth. A nursing team that had received clinical lessons in the NIDCAP approach cared for the infants in the NIDCAP intervention group. The control group in the second trial received nests to support positioning and incubator covers (basic developmental care). Parents in both groups received the support of social workers when needed, which is part of the normal protocol. The Medical Ethics Committees of both locations approved this study.

Subjects

Infants born at a gestational age (GA) below 32 weeks were randomly assigned to a control or intervention group within 48 hours after birth by using sealed envelops. Exclusion criteria were: infants of drug-addicted mothers and infants with congenital heart disease or other major birth anomalies. According to protocol, all infants admitted for less then 5 days were excluded from follow-up and analysis because the duration of the basic DC intervention was expected not to be long enough to detect an effect. A sample size power calculation showed that 140 infants (70 control, 70 intervention) were needed per RCT to show a significant difference with a power of 80%, based on the expected difference of half a standard deviation on the primary outcome of the two RCT's (developmental tests at follow up). After parental informed consent was obtained, both parents were given a questionnaire to complete at home one week after their infant's birth (after one week of admission). Infant and parent characteristics were obtained from the medical records and the questionnaire.

Measures

Infant and parent characteristics:

The infant and parent characteristics used to describe and compare the groups were: gender, gestational age (GA) at birth, birth weight, Clinical Risk Index for Babies (CRIB) score, infant's age when parents completed the questionnaire (days after birth), duration of admission to the intervention NICU, parental age, parental educational level and whether parents were living together or not. The CRIB score [20] assesses initial neonatal risk by scoring birth weight, gestational age, congenital malformation, maximal base excess in the first 12 hours and minimum and maximal oxygen requirements in the first 12 hours after birth.

Mothers and Baby Scale (MABS):

Two scales of the Mothers and Baby Scale [21] were used and translated into Dutch, being the Confidence in Caregiving (CC) scale (α=0.93; 13 items) and the Global Confidence (GC) scale (α=0.78; 3 items). Some items were slightly altered to make them more appropriate for the NICU setting. For example, the item "I've been afraid I might drop my baby" was changed into "I've been afraid that I might accidentally pull one of the lines or tubes loose". The reliability of the scales was reasonable in the present study (CC mother/father α=0.80/0.78, GC mother/father α=0.63/0.60). Items were recoded before analysis so that all item categories were on a 6-point Likert scale ranging from 0 (very insecure) to 5 (very confident) with a higher score corresponding with higher parental confidence.

Nurse Parent Support Tool (NPST):

The Nurse Parent Support Tool [22], consists of 21 descriptions of nurse support on a 5-point Likert scale ranging from 1 (almost never seen) to 5 (almost always seen) and a total nurse support scale (α=0.95) measuring the amount of nurse support parents perceive. Examples of items are: "The nursing staff at this hospital in general has: ...Taught me how to take care of my child" or "...Made me feel important as the parent". A higher score corresponded with higher perceived nurse support. The Cronbach's alpha of this translated Dutch version was 0.90 (for mothers) and 0.92 (for fathers).

Parental Stressor Scale-NICU (PSS-NICU):
The Parental Stressor Scale-NICU [23] includes 44 descriptions of NICU related stressors and 1 item concerning the overall stress of parents, all on a 5-point Likert scale ranging from 1 (not stressful) to 5 (very stressful). There is an extra answer possibility for parents to indicate that they did not experience the stressor (not applicable), which was assigned a score of 1 (not stressful). The questionnaire consists of five subscales measuring parental stress on: infant's appearance, parent role alterations, sights and sounds, staff behavior and communication and a total score. The infant's appearance scale includes stressors such as; "tubes and equipment on or near my baby" and "when my baby seemed to be in pain". The parent role alterations scale includes stressors such as; "being separated from my baby", "not being able to hold my baby when I want" and "feeling helpless about how to help my baby". A higher score corresponded with a higher stress level. Alpha reliability scores ranged from 0.73 to 0.96 [23-25]. In the present study, using the Dutch translation, the alpha scale reliability for the total score scale was 0.93 (alpha scores for the scales ranged from 0.72 to 0.89).

Analysis
For statistical analysis SPSS 11.0 for Windows was used. Average scale scores were calculated if the scale contained no more than 30% missing items. To test whether the infant and parent characteristics at birth were comparable between groups, the Chi square test, the Chi-square test for trend, the two-sample t-test or the non-parametric Mann-Whitney test were applied where appropriate.

To measure effect size between groups a covariance analysis was carried out in which some of the infant and parent characteristics (the infant's gender, GA at birth, CRIB score, parental age, parental educational level and the infant's age when parents completed the questionnaire) were included as covariates. This was done to obtain a more precise estimation of the differences between the intervention and control groups. The differences between mother and father per infant were also compared between groups with a covariance analysis. Because of multiple testing a p-value of below 0.01 was chosen to indicate significance on all outcomes.

Results

Subjects

The loss to follow-up and return rates of both RCT's are shown in Figure 1. The loss to follow-up in this figure also includes infants transferred within 5 days of admission.

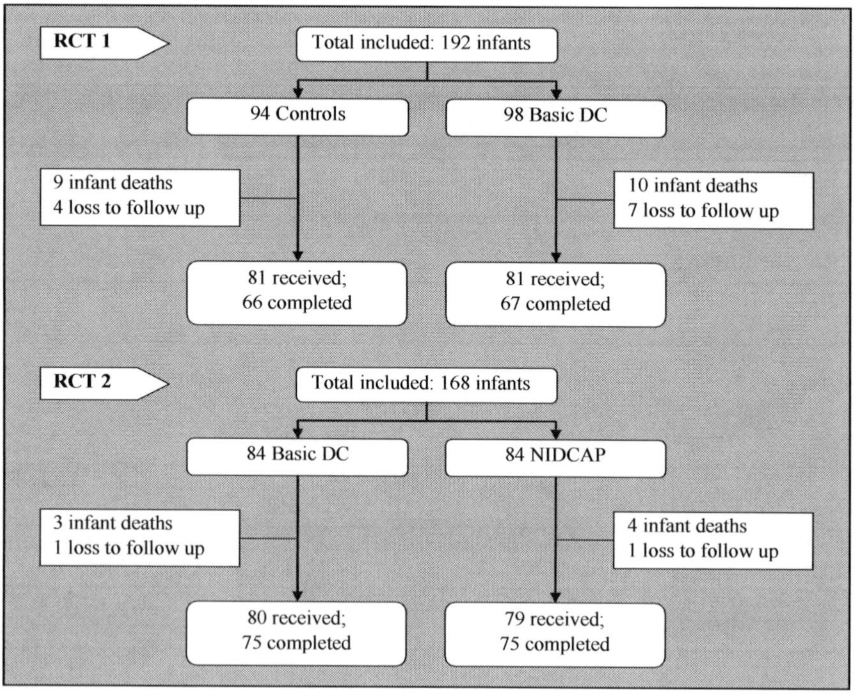

Figure 1. Loss to follow up and returned questionnaires.

During the first RCT, 133 questionnaires were returned (82% of the 162 sets of parents that were given the questionnaire and 77% of all included infants minus deaths). One mother and 6 fathers in the standard care control group and 1 mother and 3 fathers in the basic DC intervention group did not complete the questionnaires while their spouse did.

During the second RCT 150 questionnaires were returned (94% of 159 parents that received the questionnaire and 93% of all included infants minus deaths). Two mothers and 2 fathers in the basic DC control group and 7 fathers in the NIDCAP intervention group in the second trial did not complete the questionnaires while their spouse did.

The two groups in the first RCT were comparable regarding the parent characteristics (Table 1). The two groups in the second RCT were comparable regarding the child characteristics but mothers in the NIDCAP group tended to be younger (p=.02). This variable was included as one of the covariates in the covariance analysis. The infants in both groups during both trials whose parents did not receive (because of loss or death) or complete the questionnaire, were also comparable concerning gender, gestational age at birth and birth weight (data not shown).

		Controls (N=66)	Basic DC (N=67)	Basic DC (N=75)	NIDCAP (N=75)
		mean(sd) or n(%) ^	mean(sd) or n(%) ^	mean(sd) or n(%) ^	mean(sd) or n(%) ^
Gender (male), n(%)		42 (64%)	32 (48%)	37 (49%)	43 (57%)
Gestational age at birth (weeks)		28.9 (1.9)	29.0 (1.7)	29.3 (1.6)	29.6 (1.7)
Birth weight (grams)		1185 (341)	1193 (329)	1247 (344)	1239 (319)
CRIB score[2]		4.1 (3.0)	4.0 (3.8)	2.8 (3.0)	2.9 (2.8)
Both parents caucasian, n(%)		52 (84%)	49 (75%)	59 (82%)	56 (78%)
Parents not living together, n(%)		4 (6%)	4 (6%)	4 (5%)	9 (12%)
Maternal age (years), n(%)	**<25**	7 (11%)	13 (19%)	4 (5%)*	11 (15%)*
	25-35	47 (71%)	38 (57%)	47 (63%)	49 (65%)
	>35	12 (18%)	16 (24%)	24 (32%)	15 (20%)
Maternal educational level[1]	**Low**	18 (27%)	24 (36%)	18 (24%)	26 (36%)
n(%)	**Interm.**	31 (47%)	27 (41%)	25 (34%)	25 (35%)
	High	17 (26%)	15 (23%)	31 (42%)	21 (29%)
Paternal age (years), n(%)	**<25**	5 (8%)	4 (6%)	4 (5%)	4 (5%)
	25-35	31 (47%)	35 (53%)	39 (53%)	52 (69%)
	>35	30 (46%)	27 (41%)	31 (42%)	19 (25%)
Paternal educational level[1]	**Low**	20 (30%)	22 (33%)	15 (21%)	19 (28%)
n(%)	**Interm.**	26 (39%)	25 (38%)	31 (43%)	22 (32%)
	High	20 (30%)	19 (29%)	27 (37%)	28 (41%)
Infant's age completion questionnaire (days) #		10 (6-29)	11 (6-67)	14 (4-85)	14 (6-88)
Admission duration (days) #		34 (5-105)	40 (6-142)	30 (5-128)	38 (6-160)

Table 1. Comparison of infant and parent characteristics of returned questionnaire.

* sign. p-value < .05
1 educational level: low (vocational training) / intermediate (high school) / high (college education/ university)
2 Clinical Risk Index for Babies (CRIB), [20]
^ statistical tests used : chi-square test (for linear trend), n(%) / two-sample t-test, mean(sd)
\# non parametric Mann-Whitney test, median (range).

Effect of basic developmental care and NIDCAP

No significant differences were found on mother's confidence, perceived nursing support and stress scores in both trials (Table 2). The expected decrease in maternal stress in both trials and increase in maternal confidence and perceived nurse support of the mothers in the NIDCAP group in the second trial were not found. Mothers in the basic DC intervention group during the first trial tended to show more stress on the subscale staff behavior and communication (p=.05), compared to the standard care controls.

The scores of fathers in both RCT's also did not show significant differences and the expected effects were not observed (Table 2). Fathers in the NIDCAP intervention group in the second trial reported more stress on the subscale staff behavior and communication, but this difference was not significant (p=.046). In the first trial the fathers in the basic DC intervention group also tended to experience more stress compared to the standard care control group (NS).

In both trials, overall mean parental confidence scores were approximately 3.50, which corresponds with being moderately confident. Mean nurse support scores were approximately 4.30, which corresponds with nursing staff showing much support. Mean stressor scores were approximately 2.00, which corresponds with NICU stressors being a little stressful.

Effect on difference between father and mother

Overall, the largest differences in stress level between mother and father were on the PSS-NICU subscale parent role alterations. No significant effects of the two interventions were found on the difference of mothers and fathers regarding parental confidence, perceived nurse support and parental stress in both trials (Table 3). The difference in total stress levels of mothers (higher) compared to fathers tended to be lower in the NIDCAP intervention group in the second RCT (p=.034).

	Controls	Basic DC	RCT 1	Basic DC	NIDCAP	RCT 2
Mother Total scales ~	**Mean (sd)**	**Mean (sd)**	**Diff (99%CI)#**	**Mean (sd)**	**Mean (sd)**	**Diff (99%CI)#**
Confidence caregiving	3.46 (.72)	3.41 (.75)	.09 (-.27;.44)	3.34 (.76)	3.43 (.65)	-.09 (-.42;.23)
Global confidence	3.42 (.86)	3.41 (.94)	.03 (-.40;.46)	3.39 (.80)	3.49 (.78)	.01 (-.35;.36)
Nurse support	4.19 (.54)	4.18 (.52)	.04 (-.21;.29)	4.14 (.51)	4.26 (.53)	-.14 (-.37;.10)
Total stressor score	2.09 (.55)	2.16 (.58)	-.12 (-.38;.15)	2.25 (.60)	2.16 (.54)	.09 (-.18;.36)
Father Total scales ~	**Mean (sd)**	**Mean (sd)**	**Diff (99%CI)#**	**Mean (sd)**	**Mean (sd)**	**Diff (99%CI)#**
Confidence caregiving	3.46 (.62)	3.43 (.69)	.06 (-.27;.39)	3.51 (.70)	3.45 (.65)	.05 (-.27;.36)
Global confidence	3.73 (.80)	3.67 (.93)	.05 (-.37;.46)	3.79 (.73)	3.67 (.77)	.10 (-.24;.44)
Nurse support	4.10 (.57)	4.21 (.56)	-.10 (-.37;.18)	4.17 (.48)	4.23 (.58)	-.07 (-.30;.17)
Total stressor score	1.88 (.45)	1.98 (.59)	-.11 (-.37;.15)	1.85 (.55)	2.05 (.57)	-.15 (-.40;.10)
PSS stressor subscale:						
Staff behav & comm.	*1.42 (.57)*	*1.56 (.66)*	*-.10 (-.41;.21)*	*1.34 (.59)*	*1.55 (.77)*	*-.25 (-.56;.07)**

Table 2. Effect of basic elements of developmental care on parental stress, confidence and perceived nurse support.

* p-value < .05

~ higher mean score represents: higher confidence, higher nurse support, higher stress levels

\# differences (C-DC and DC-NIDCAP) after adjusting for covariates (infant and parent characteristics being; gender, GA at birth, CRIB score, day of completing the questionnaire, parental age and parental educational level). Min N on total scales C1; mother=61, father=58, I1; mother=60, father=60, C2; mother=66, father=67, I2; mother=68, father=63

	Controls	Basic DC	RCT 1	Basic DC	NIDCAP	RCT 2
	Mean (sd)	Mean (sd)	Diff (99%CI)#	Mean (sd)	Mean (sd)	Diff (99%CI)#
Confidence caregiving	.052 (.67)	-.002 (.68)	.11 (-.23;.46)	-.161 (.77)	.012 (.56)	-.16 (-.49;.18)
Global confidence	-.328 (.74)	-.280 (.85)	.04 (-.35;.43)	-.376 (.93)	-.211 (1.01)	-.09 (-.57;.39)
Nurse support	.103 (.51)	-.020 (.48)	.17 (-.08;.42)	-.024 (.51)	-.006 (.52)	-.01 (-.26;.25)
Total stressor score	.199 (.60)	.183 (.56)	-.04 (-.33;.25)	.410 (.57)	.142 (.57)	.23 (-.05;.50)*
PSS stressor subscales:						
Sights and sounds	*.305 (.74)*	*.118 (.77)*	*.17 (-.21;.54)*	*.379 (.68)*	*.159 (.71)*	*.18 (-.15;.51)*
Infant's appearance	*.174 (.89)*	*.163 (.81)*	*-.09 (-.51;.33)*	*.447 (.76)*	*.184 (.66)*	*.23 (-.11;.57)*
Parent role alterations	*.438 (.76)*	*.374 (.73)*	*.04 (-.35;.42)*	*.621 (.78)*	*.331 (.96)*	*.24 (-.18;.65)*
Staff behav & comm.	*-.088 (.46)*	*.033 (.70)*	*-.17 (-.47;.14)*	*.172 (.76)*	*-.061 (.70)*	*.21 (-.16;58)*

Table 3. Difference between mother and father (if both completed the questionnaire).

* p-value < .05, paired t-test

\# differences (C-DC and DC-NIDCAP) after adjusting for covariates (infant and parent characteristics being; gender, GA at birth, CRIB score, day of completing the questionnaire, parental age and parental educational level). Min N on total scales C1=56, I1=59, C2=65, I2=62

Discussion

During two randomized controlled trials, measuring first the effect of the basics elements of developmental care compared to standard care and secondly the effect of NIDCAP compared to basic DC, no effects were found of developmental care and NIDCAP on parental confidence, perceived nurse support and parental stress of mothers and fathers of very preterm infants during admission. The differences found between groups were mostly small in both trials.

Overall, mothers in this study reported more stress compared to fathers. This difference tended to decrease in the NIDCAP intervention group in the second trial, but this was mainly caused by a higher stress level of the fathers in the NIDCAP intervention group. A higher parental stress level of mothers compared to fathers, as found in the current study, has previously been found and explored in other studies [18,19,26,27]. Miles et al. suggested that because mothers score highest on "parent role alteration" stressors, they are more affected by the loss of the caretaking role [27]. This large difference in stress between mother and father on parent role alterations was also found in the current study. Jackson et al. [26] examined the difference in experiences of both father and mother more extensively. Mothers felt a need to participate more in the caregiving of their infant and some mothers felt they were "borrowing their child from the staff" leading to feelings of insecurity. Fathers expressed the feeling of being an outsider because of the preterm delivery, but some had difficulty getting leave from work and had no choice but to leave the care to the staff [26].

In the current study, the difference in stress levels of mothers compared to fathers was lower (but not significantly) in the NIDCAP intervention group compared to the basic developmental care control group. Studies up to date have mainly focused on maternal stress. The effect of increased paternal stress on the preterm infant and the family due to the effects of NIDCAP on the stress levels of fathers have not been studied yet, to our knowledge. Pierrehumbert et al. [7] found that both maternal and paternal post-traumatic reactions increased infant sleeping and eating problems reported by parents.

The lower difference of maternal and parental stress levels in the NIDCAP group, although non-significant, might be caused by a more active involvement of fathers during the NIDCAP guidance. This might result in paternal stress levels that are more comparable with maternal stress levels. This study shows that future research exploring the effects of early intervention in the neonatal intensive care unit needs to focus on the involvement and stress levels of fathers.
The effect of the NIDCAP intervention on parents has previously been examined in a three-center RCT by Als et al. [11]. This study found less parental stress on the total child and parent domain scales and the total score of the Parent Stress Index (PSI) at two weeks after the expected date of confinement following the NIDCAP intervention with infants born < 28 weeks of gestation and weighing < 1250 grams. Furthermore, mothers perceived their children as more independent individuals on the Mother's View of the Child (MVC) [11]. A recent NIDCAP study with 20 mothers by Kleberg et al. [16] concluded that although mothers in the NIDCAP group perceived more nurse support and closeness to their infant, they also expressed more anxiety. The authors suggested that higher anxiety might be a sign of early bonding [16]. A recent Dutch study [28] concluded that parents of infants born <30 weeks of gestation receiving NIDCAP were significantly more satisfied with the caregiving and parents indicated more nurse support on the NPST questionnaire but, as in the current study, this difference was not significant. Other intervention studies, mainly based on coping and stress of parents of preterm born infants, used the parental PSS-NICU questionnaire and did show positive results [29,30].

Parents in this study indicated little stress (an average score of 2) on the stressors stated in the PSS-NICU. In other studies the stress scores appeared to be somewhat higher, with mean values of 2.5 to 3.0 [25,27,30]. Two recent studies [24,29] also found mean total scores of approximately 2. Parental age and infant birth weight and gestation in these studies were comparable to the present study. Mean perceived nurse support scores ranged from 4.13 to 4.27, which indicated that parents are in general satisfied with the support shown by the nursing staff. In a previous Dutch NIDCAP study [28] NPST scores were comparable (mean score of 4.10 for controls and 4.26 for the NIDCAP

intervention group). These scores do not leave much of a window of opportunity to decrease parental stress and improve nurse support. Furthermore, prenatal and neonatal care and the support from social workers in the Netherlands is equally available for all people from different social economic backgrounds, which might lead to moderate stress levels and relatively high perceived nurse support in general.
The questionnaires were given after one week of admission because some children were already transferred to a regional hospital by then. In the Netherlands, infants receive intensive care at an academic unit and are transferred to a regional hospital once they become more stable. The questionnaires were on average completed in the second week of admission (Table 1). One or two weeks of intervention might not be an adequate amount of time to already measure effect on parents' experiences at the unit. In the second trial on average only one or two NIDCAP observations were done when parents completed the questionnaire. However, at that moment, parents were experiencing strong emotions regarding the preterm birth and the sudden admission of their infant in the intensive care unit. They might feel the need for guidance most during the first weeks of admission and the outcomes measured (parental stressors in the unit and perceived nurse support) related to parental experiences during the admission of their infant in the unit. Furthermore, the intervention already started within 48 hours after birth.

The return rates of this study were good, which implies that the research sample provided a good representation of all infants below 32 weeks admitted to a Dutch NICU. Other outcome variables of this study, related to the infant's medical condition and outcomes at follow-up, will be presented in the future.

In conclusion, both basic developmental care and the complete NIDCAP care program with individual observations and guidance had no significant effect on perceived nurse support, parental stress and parental confidence. The expected effect of a decrease in parental stress of both interventions and the expected positive effect of the NIDCAP intervention on parental confidence and perceived nurse support was not observed. As a result of increased paternal stress, the NIDCAP intervention tended to decrease the difference in stress levels of fathers and mothers. The NIDCAP program may therefore lead to increased involvement of fathers, compared to a basic form of developmental care, leading to more comparable stress levels of fathers and mothers.

Acknowledgements

We are grateful to the parents for taking the time and effort to fill in the questionnaires. We would also like to thank the medical and nursing staff at the Leiden University Medical Center, especially dr. S. Veen for her assistance, and the Juliana Children's Hospital, especially dr. P. van Zwieten and dr. A. Sprij, for their involvement in this study. We are also indebted to the NIDCAP-trained nurses. We furthermore thank ZONMW (grant 2100.0072) and the Health Care Efficiency Research Fund LUMC for funding this study.

References

1. Lau,R. & Morse,C.A. Stress experiences of parents with premature infants in a special care nursery. *Stress and Health* **19**, 69-78 (2003).

2. Singer,L.T. *et al.* Maternal psychological distress and parenting stress after the birth of a very low-birth-weight infant. *JAMA* **281**, 799-805 (1999).

3. Rautava,P., Lehtonen,L., Helenius,H. & Sillanpaa,M. Effect of newborn hospitalization on family and child behavior: a 12-year follow-up study. *Pediatrics* **111**, 277-283 (2003).

4. Holditch-Davis,D., Bartlett,T.R., Blickman,A.L. & Miles,M.S. Posttraumatic stress symptoms in mothers of premature infants. *J. Obstet. Gynecol. Neonatal Nurs.* **32**, 161-171 (2003).

5. Allen,E.C. *et al.* Perception of child vulnerability among mothers of former premature infants. *Pediatrics* **113**, 267-273 (2004).

6. Miceli,P.J. *et al.* Brief report: birth status, medical complications, and social environment: individual differences in development of preterm, very low birth weight infants. *J. Pediatr. Psychol.* **25**, 353-358 (2000).

7. Pierrehumbert,B., Nicole,A., Muller-Nix,C., Forcada-Guex,M. & Ansermet,F. Parental post-traumatic reactions after premature birth: implications for sleeping and eating problems in the infant. *Arch. Dis. Child Fetal Neonatal Ed* **88**, F400-F404 (2003).

8. Spear,M.L., Leef,K., Epps,S. & Locke,R. Family reactions during infants' hospitalization in the neonatal intensive care unit. *Am. J. Perinatol.* **19**, 205-213 (2002).

9. Als,H. Developmental Interventions in the Neonatal Intensive Care Nursery. Goldson,E. (ed.), pp. 18-85 (Oxford University Press, New York,1999).

10. Als,H. *et al.* Individualized developmental care for the very low-birth-weight preterm infant. Medical and neurofunctional effects. *JAMA* **272**, 853-858 (1994).

11. Als,H. *et al.* A three-center, randomized, controlled trial of individualized developmental care for very low birth weight preterm infants: medical, neurodevelopmental, parenting, and caregiving effects. *J. Dev. Behav. Pediatr.* **24**, 399-408 (2003).

12. Als,H. *et al.* Early experience alters brain function and structure. *Pediatrics* **113**, 846-857 (2004).

13. Kleberg,A., Westrup,B. & Stjernqvist,K. Developmental outcome, child behaviour and mother-child interaction at 3 years of age following Newborn Individualized Developmental Care and Intervention Program (NIDCAP) intervention. *Early Hum. Dev.* **60**, 123-135 (2000).

14. Kleberg,A., Westrup,B., Stjernqvist,K. & Lagercrantz,H. Indications of improved cognitive development at one year of age among infants born very prematurely who received care based on the Newborn Individualized Developmental Care and Assessment Program (NIDCAP). *Early Hum. Dev.* **68**, 83-91 (2002).

15. Westrup,B., Bohm,B., Lagercrantz,H. & Stjernqvist,K. Preschool outcome in children born very prematurely and cared for according to the Newborn Individualized Developmental Care and Assessment Program (NIDCAP). *Acta Paediatr.* **93**, 498-507 (2004).

16. Kleberg,A., Hellstrom-Westas,L. & Widstrom,A.M. Mothers' perception of Newborn Individualized Developmental Care and Assessment Program (NIDCAP) as compared to conventional care. *Early Hum. Dev.* (2006).

17. Symington,A. & Pinelli,J. Developmental care for promoting development and preventing morbidity in preterm infants. *Cochrane. Database. Syst. Rev.* CD001814 (2006).

18. Dudek-Shriber,L. Parent stress in the neonatal intensive care unit and the influence of parent and infant characteristics. *Am. J. Occup. Ther.* **58**, 509-520 (2004).

19. Tommiska,V., Ostberg,M. & Fellman,V. Parental stress in families of 2 year old extremely low birthweight infants. *Arch. Dis. Child Fetal Neonatal Ed* **86**, F161-F164 (2002).

20. The International Neonatal Network. The CRIB (clinical risk index for babies) score: a tool for assessing initial neonatal risk and comparing performance of neonatal intensive care units. *Lancet* **342**, 193-198 (1993).

21. Wolke,D. Neonatal Behavioral Assessment Scale, 3rd edition. Brazelton,T.B. & Nugent,J.K. (eds.), pp. 117-125 (Mac Keith Press, Cambridge,1995).

22. Miles,M.S., Carlson,J. & Brunssen,S. The nurse parent support tool. *J. Pediatr. Nurs.* **14**, 44-50 (1999).

23. Miles,M.S., Funk,S.G. & Carlson,J. Parental Stressor Scale: neonatal intensive care unit. *Nurs. Res.* **42**, 148-152 (1993).

24. Franck,L.S., Cox,S., Allen,A. & Winter,I. Measuring neonatal intensive care unit-related parental stress. *J. Adv. Nurs.* **49**, 608-615 (2005).

25. Reid,T. Using the Parental Stressor Scale: NICU with a British sample of mothers of moderate risk preterm infants. *Journal of Reproductive and Infant Psychology* **21**, 279-291 (2003).

26. Jackson,K., Ternestedt,B.M. & Schollin,J. From alienation to familiarity: experiences of mothers and fathers of preterm infants. *J. Adv. Nurs.* **43**, 120-129 (2003).

27. Miles,M.S., Funk,S.G. & Kasper,M.A. The stress response of mothers and fathers of preterm infants. *Res. Nurs. Health* **15**, 261-269 (1992).

28. Wielenga,J.M., Smit,B.J. & Unk,L.K. How satisfied are parents supported by nurses with the NIDCAP model of care for their preterm infant? *J. Nurs. Care Qual.* **21**, 41-48 (2006).

29. Melnyk,B.M. *et al.* Reducing premature infants' length of stay and improving parents' mental health outcomes with the Creating Opportunities for Parent Empowerment (COPE) neonatal intensive care unit program: a randomized, controlled trial. *Pediatrics* **118**, e1414-e1427 (2006).

30. Preyde,M. & Ardal,F. Effectiveness of a parent "buddy" program for mothers of very preterm infants in a neonatal intensive care unit. *CMAJ.* **168**, 969-973 (2003).

CHAPTER 3

Health-Related Quality of Life of very preterm infants at 1 year of age after two Developmental Care based interventions

YLVIA M. VAN DER PAL
ELESTE M. MAGUIRE
ANET BRUIL
ASKIA LE CESSIE
N MAARTEN WIT
RANS J. WALTHER
YLVIA VEEN

Abstract

Background:

In the context of a growing interest in developmental care this study explores the effect of the basic elements of developmental care (DC) and the additional effect of the individual approach of the Newborn Individualized Developmental Care and Assessment Program (NIDCAP®) on health-related quality of life (HRQoL) of very preterm infants at 1 year of age. The basic elements of Developmental Care in this study were defined as the use of standardized nests and incubator covers, whose protective characteristics were hypothesized to have a positive effect on the infant's health-related quality of life. The individualized approach of the NIDCAP was thought to further increase HRQoL.

Methods:

Very preterm (≤ 32 weeks) born infants in a Dutch Neonatal Intensive Care Unit at two locations were included in two consecutive randomized controlled trials (RCT) comparing controls (standard care) versus basic developmental care (standardized nests and covers) in the first RCT and basic developmental care versus NIDCAP in the second RCT. Parents completed a questionnaire (RCT1 n=136, RCT2 n=128) regarding their infant's HRQoL (TAPQoL) at 1 year of age, corrected for prematurity. Because of multiple testing a p-value of below 0.01 was chosen to indicate significance.

Results:

HRQoL scores were good to optimal for most infants. No significant differences were found between basic DC versus controls and NIDCAP versus basic DC on the child's HRQoL at 1 year of age, as reported by parents

Conclusion:

These two randomized controlled trials show that the basic elements of Developmental Care and the more individualized NIDCAP do not improve health-related quality of life of very preterm infants at 1 year of age.

Introduction

Advances in neonatology have decreased the mortality of infants born very preterm [1,2] and neonatal caregiving in the Neonatal Intensive Care Unit (NICU) has shifted towards a more family-centered and individualized approach. In the 1980's Als introduced the Newborn Individualized Developmental Care and Assessment Program (NIDCAP) [3] in the NICU. This program is based on the Synactive Theory of Development where the preterm infant's individual behavior and efforts at self-regulation are observed through approach and avoidance behaviors by a trained developmental specialist [4]. Recommendations to support the infant and family are made based on these observations and are discussed with parents and other caregivers [3,5].

A recent Cochrane review on Developmental Care [6] concluded that positive effects of NIDCAP on short-term health outcomes during admission regarding moderate-severe lung disease and incidence of necrotizing enterocolitis. This review however also concluded that the significant effects were mainly based on studies with small sample sizes and several of these findings were not supported in other settings [6]. Furthermore, the studies only reported on short-term health outcomes and there was no mention of studies done to evaluate the effect of NIDCAP on health outcomes after discharge.

Implementing NIDCAP by training nurses to administer the observational tool and implementing the individualized care is costly and time-consuming. As a result hospitals may primarily focus on the basic elements of developmental care programs. Basic elements of developmental care (DC) programs are, for example, the use of standardized incubator covers to reduce light and the use of standardized nests for positioning and to support motor development and physiological stability. These basic elements focus on protecting the infant from intense environmental stimuli and on promoting self-soothing behaviors, motor development, physical stability and health.

Quality of life has become an important outcome measure of neonatal care, in addition to mortality and morbidity. This has led to the development of questionnaires to monitor the infant's health-related quality of life (HRQoL) [7]. HRQoL is defined as the functioning of the child on four dimensions: physical functioning, social functioning, cognitive functioning and emotional functioning, weighted by the emotional evaluation of the problems [8,9]. In previous studies very preterm children showed lower scores compared to reference groups of children born at term on several scales of HRQoL questionnaires [10-13].

The current study was designed to measure whether the use of the basic elements of developmental care would improve health-related quality of life of very preterm infants. The additional effect of the more intensive and individualized NIDCAP program compared to basic developmental care, on health-related quality of life, was explored in a second randomized controlled trial. The effect of developmental care on HRQoL has, to our knowledge, not yet been studied. Our hypothesis was that application of the basic elements of developmental care would increase health-related quality of life after 1 year because of the protective properties of the covers from environmental stimuli and the support of the standardized nests on the infant's self-soothing behaviors, motor development and physiological stability. Secondly, the individual NIDCAP program was thought to further increase HRQoL because this program is even more focused on creating opportunities for the infant to rest and recover.

Methods

The first randomized controlled trial (inclusion April 2000 – May 2002) measured the effect of basic Developmental Care (DC) versus standard nursing care. The intervention was based on the reduction of light and sound through the use of standardized incubator covers and on supporting motor development and physiological stability by positioning the infant in ways that encourage flexion and containment through the use of standardized nests. The control (C) group received standard care prior to this study, when no incubator covers or forms of nesting were used.

The second randomized controlled trial (inclusion July 2002 to August 2004) studied the additional effect of the individual approach of NIDCAP compared to the basic elements of developmental care. The intervention in the second trial consisted of basic developmental care and NIDCAP observations of the infant before, during and after caregiving [3] every 7 to 10 days by a NIDCAP-trained developmental specialist. The trained developmental specialist wrote reports and discussed individualized recommendations with parents and other caregivers and supported them in giving care to the infant. The first observation was done within 48 hours after birth. A nursing team that received additional clinical lessons in the NIDCAP approach was assigned to the infants in the NIDCAP invention group. The control group in the second trial was given nests to support positioning and incubator covers (basic developmental care).

Subjects

In both trials, infants born with a gestational age below 32 weeks admitted to a NICU at two locations in the Netherlands, were randomly assigned (cards in sealed envelops) to a control group (first RCT: control standard care, second RCT: basic DC) or intervention group (first RCT: basic DC, second RCT: NIDCAP) within 48 hours after birth.

Exclusion criteria were: infants of drug-addicted mothers and infants with congenital heart disease or other major birth anomalies. According to protocol, infants in both groups who were admitted for less then 5 days were excluded from the follow-up of the current study because the duration of the basic DC intervention was hypothesized to be too short. After parental informed consent was obtained, 192 infants were included.

During outpatient clinic visits at 1 year of age, corrected for prematurity, the TNO-AZL Preschool Quality of Life Questionnaire (TAPQoL for infants under 18 months of age) [14], was given to parents to complete at home. All ages mentioned hereafter are corrected for prematurity. The Medical Ethics Committees of both locations approved this study.

Measures

Parent and child characteristics:

Demographic variables included parental age, educational level and country of birth (the Netherlands/other). Infant characteristics at birth were the infant's gender, gestational age, birth weight and the Clinical Risk Index for Babies (CRIB) score. The CRIB score [15] assesses initial neonatal risk by scoring birth weight, gestational age, congenital malformation, maximal base excess value (a measure of metabolic acidosis secondary to hypoxia) in the first 12 hours and minimum and maximal oxygen requirements in the first 12 hours after birth.

HRQoL (TAPQoL) questionnaire:

The TNO-AZL Preschool Quality of Life Questionnaire 35 item version (TAPQoL) [14,16] was used. The TAPQoL is a multidimensional instrument for children 0-5 years of age with the following HRQoL scales; stomach, skin, lungs, sleeping, appetite, liveliness, positive mood, problem behavior, anxiety, motor functioning, social functioning and communication. An additional scale measuring eating problems for children born preterm was used as well. For children under 18 months of age the scales motor functioning, social functioning and communication do not apply.

The frequency of a specific complaint or limitation during the last three months was recorded first (for example: "In the last 3 months, has your child experienced any stomach or belly pain: never / occasionally / often"). If parents reported a problem, they were asked to rate the well-being of the child in relation to this problem (fine, not so good, quite bad or bad). Each item was encoded into one single score, ranging from 0 to 4 (4= no problem, 3= child has a problem (occasionally or often) but feels fine, 2= child has a problem and feels not so well, 1= child has a problem and feels quite bad, 0= child has a problem and feels bad). The scales measuring problem behavior, anxiety, positive mood and liveliness, did not ask how the child felt since the items already implied a positive or negative emotional state (for example: "my child was angry") and scores are 0 (often), 1 (occasionally) or 2 (never). All item scores were transformed to a scale score ranging from 0 to 100 with a higher score indicating a better HRQoL. In previous studies [13,14,17] the

TAPQoL showed good validity and reliability with Cronbach's alpha reliability scores ranging from respectively 0.66 to 0.88 for Dutch preterm infants. In the current study alpha reliability scores ranged from 0.50 to 0.91.

Analysis

SPSS 11.0 for Windows was used for statistical analysis. To test whether the infant and parent characteristics were comparable between groups, the Chi square test, the Chi-square test for trend, the two-sample t-test or the non-parametric Mann-Whitney test were applied where appropriate.

The TAPQoL scales were skewed, with most infants receiving an optimal HRQoL score of 100 (ceiling effect). Therefore, scores where divided into categories of <70 (non-optimal), 70-99 (sub-optimal) and 100 (optimal) and the percentage of infants scoring within a category was reported, as described in an earlier Dutch study using the TAPQoL [12]. Chi-square tests for linear trend were performed to compare the percentages scoring in the categories on the HRQoL scales for both groups in both RCT's. Because of multiple testing a p-value of below 0.01 was chosen to indicate significance. An overall main effect of the groups was calculated with a multivariate analysis with all TAPQoL scales scores as dependent variables.

Results

Subjects

During the first RCT 192 infants were included. At 1 year 143 parents received the questionnaire of which 136 (95%) were returned (Figure 1). The return rate of all 192 included children minus 25 infant deaths was 81%. During the second RCT 168 infants were included. At 1 year 144 parents received the questionnaire of which 128 (89%) were returned (Figure 1). The return rate of all 168 included children minus 14 infant deaths was 83%. Loss to follow-up also included infants transferred within 5 days of admission.

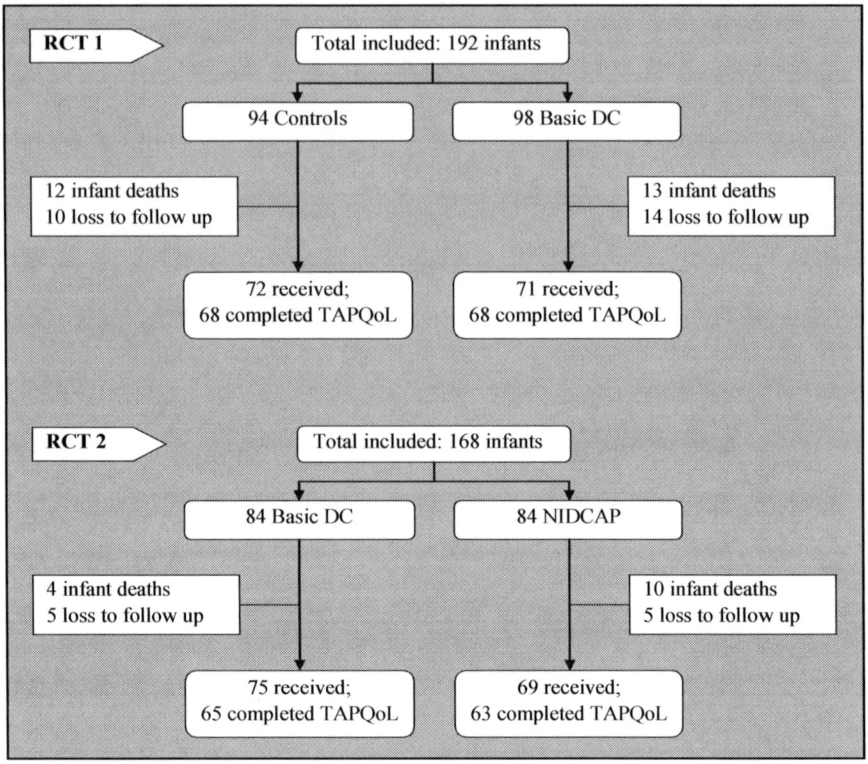

Figure 1. Loss to follow up and returned questionnaires.

The infant and parent characteristics of the parents who returned the questionnaire at 1 year were similar in both groups (Table 1), with the exception of maternal age (p=0.007), which was lower in the NIDCAP intervention group. However, mothers in both groups were on average in their thirties and their educational levels did not differ significantly and therefore maternal age was not expected to be a confounding variable.

Basic developmental care and health-related quality of life

In the first trial, no significant differences between the standard care control and basic DC intervention group were found on the TAPQoL scale scores (Table 2). For the scale 'appetite' HRQoL tended to be more often optimal in the DC group. However, for most scales (stomach, skin, lungs, eating disorders, and problem behavior) HRQoL more often tended to be optimal in the control group compared to the basic DC group. The main effect of basic DC on all scale scores was not significant (p=0.84).

Table 1. Comparison of infant and parent characteristics of completed questionnaires.

		Controls (N=68) Mean(sd) or n(%)^	Basic DC (N=68) mean(sd) or n(%)^	Basic DC (N=65) mean(sd) or n(%)^	NIDCAP (N=63) mean(sd) or n(%)^
Completed by..	**mother**	47 (71%)	48 (72%)	57 (89%)	50 (79%)
	father	9 (14%)	8 (12%)	5 (8%)	9 (14%)
	both	10 (15%)	11 (16%)	2 (3%)	4 (6%)
Gender (male)		46 (68%)	37 (54%)	33 (51%)	38 (60%)
Gestational age at birth (weeks)		29.1 (1.9)	29.5 (1.6)	29.2 (1.6)	29.6 (1.5)
Birth weight (grams)		1231 (323)	1245 (345)	1244 (349)	1269 (318)
CRIB score [1]		3.7 (3.0)	3.2 (3.0)	3.0 (3.1)	2.8 (2.8)
Maternal age when completing questionn. (yrs)		31.6 (4.8)	31.2 (5.1)	33.5 (4.9) *	31.1 (5.1) *
Maternal educational level [2]	**low**	21 (31%)	29 (43%)	12 (19%)	17 (27)
	interm.	28 (42%)	23 (34%)	26 (41%)	24 (38)
	high	18 (27%)	16 (24%)	26 (41%)	22 (35)
Country of birth mother (the Netherlands)		52 (76%)	46 (68%)	58 (91%)	51 (81%)
Paternal age when completing questionn. (yrs)		34.8 (5.6)	34.2 (5.4)	35.1 (5.5)	33.3 (5.8)
Paternal educational level [2]	**low**	16 (24%)	27 (40%)	9 (15%)	12 (20%)
	interm.	30 (46%)	25 (37%)	32 (52%)	20 (34%)
	high	20 (30%)	15 (22%)	21 (34%)	27 (46%)
Country of birth father (the Netherlands)		54 (79%)	50 (74%)	50 (78%)	48 (77%)
Completing day after age 1 year (days) #		9 (-11;117)	14 (-12;95)	15 (-42;101)	10 (-35;119)
Admission duration intervention NICU (days) #		35 (5;114)	41 (6;142)	36 (5;286)	38 (6;160)

* $p < .01$

^ T-test / Chi square test (for trend)

\# Non parametric Mann-Whitney test

1 Clinical Risk Index for Babies (CRIB) [15]

2 Low = vocational education, intermediate = high school, high = college education/ university

TAPQoL scale score	**< 70, n(%)**		**70-99, n(%)**		**100, n(%)**		
RCT 1 (standard care – basic DC)	**C**	**DC**	**C**	**DC**	**C**	**DC**	**p ^**
Stomach	7 (10)	9 (13)	12 (18)	20 (30)	49 (72)	38 (57)	.13
Skin	3 (5)	8 (12)	30 (45)	33 (49)	34 (51)	27 (40)	.09
Lungs	19 (28)	21 (31)	13 (19)	16 (24)	36 (53)	31 (46)	.49
Sleeping	21 (31)	20 (29)	30 (44)	30 (44)	17 (25)	18 (27)	.82
Appetite	9 (13)	9 (13)	28 (41)	22 (32)	31 (46)	37 (54)	.47
Eating problems	5 (7)	9 (13)	25 (37)	25 (37)	38 (56)	34 (50)	.31
Liveliness	7 (10)	4 (6)	2 (3)	4 (6)	58 (87)	60 (88)	.53
Positive mood	4 (6)	6 (9)	5 (7)	3 (4)	59 (87)	59 (87)	.76
Problem behavior	8 (12)	14 (21)	48 (71)	47 (69)	12 (18)	7 (10)	.09
Anxiety	22 (32)	19 (28)	16 (24)	22 (32)	30 (44)	27 (40)	1.00
Main effect HRQoL RCT 1 ~							**.84**
RCT 2 (basic DC – NIDCAP)	**DC**	**NIDCAP**	**DC**	**NIDCAP**	**DC**	**NIDCAP**	**p ^**
Stomach	9 (14)	8 (13)	22 (34)	16 (26)	34 (52)	37 (61)	.48
Skin	3 (5)	5 (8)	27 (42)	20 (32)	35 (54)	37 (60)	.83
Lungs	17 (27)	14 (23)	14 (22)	10 (16)	33 (52)	37 (61)	.40
Sleeping	23 (35)	24 (38)	29 (45)	27 (43)	13 (20)	12 (19)	.78
Appetite	10 (15)	3 (5)	26 (40)	28 (44)	29 (45)	32 (51)	.15
Eating problems	4 (6)	4 (6)	26 (40)	19 (30)	35 (54)	40 (64)	.38
Liveliness	1 (2)	4 (6)	1 (2)	4 (6)	63 (97)	55 (87)	.06
Positive mood	2 (3)	5 (8)	2 (3)	2 (3)	61 (94)	55 (89)	.24
Problem behavior	18 (28)	18 (29)	38 (59)	34 (54)	9 (14)	11 (18)	.81
Anxiety	24 (37)	31 (49)	17 (26)	9 (14)	24 (37)	23 (37)	.42
Main effect HRQoL RCT 2 ~							**.48**

Table 2. Comparison of HRQoL scores RCT 1 (standard care - basic DC) and RCT 2 (basic DC – NIDCAP)

^ Chi square test for trend for Controls (C) versus Intervention group (I)

~ Main effect: Multivariate analysis, Hotelling's trace

NIDCAP and health-related quality of life

In the second trial, no significant differences between the basic DC control and NIDCAP intervention group were found on the TAPQoL scale scores (Table 2) and the differences that were found were small. HRQoL scores tended to be more often optimal in the NIDCAP intervention group for most scales (stomach, skin, lungs, appetite, eating disorders and problem behavior). HRQoL tended to be less often optimal in the NIDCAP intervention group for the scales liveliness and positive mood. The main effect of NIDCAP on all HRQoL scales together was non-significant (p=0.48).

Discussion

This study found no significant effects of either a basic form of developmental care (the use of standardized nest and incubator covers) or the individualized NIDCAP intervention (with individual behavior observations and guidance) on health-related quality of life at 1 year of age during two consecutive RCT's with a large sample of Dutch preterm infants. In the first RCT, the small differences of basic developmental care compared to standard care showed no pattern of effect. The hypothesis that the protection of covers and the positioning support of nests might give children more rest and support during admission and as a result might have led to improved health-related quality of life is therefore not supported by the results of this study. In the second RCT also only small non-significant differences were found which does not support the hypothesis that the more individualized care would further increase HRQoL in addition to basic DC.

The design of the current study, with two consecutive trials, made it possible to explore the effect of a basic DC intervention and the additional effect of a more individualized intervention. However, a side effect of this design is that it becomes difficult to compare the standard care controls in the first RCT with the infants receiving the individualized NIDCAP in the second RCT, which took place two years later. Furthermore, the average HRQoL scores of the infants in the two basic DC groups in both trials, who received the same intervention, often differed.

While a recent Cochrane review on Developmental Care [6] reported some positive effects of NIDCAP on short term health outcomes during admission there was no mention of studies evaluating the effect of NIDCAP on health outcomes after discharge. A study regarding the effect of the Infant Health and Development Program, a longitudinal home visit intervention until 3 years of age, found no effects on serious health conditions and an increase in reported minor illnesses within the lower birth weight infants in their intervention group when the intervention ended at 3 years of age. The authors suggested that this might be due to reporting bias by mothers and the more intense health surveillance and education in the intervention group. They found no effect on health outcomes reported by parents at 5 and 8 years of age [18-20].

Parents in our study were asked to give an impression of their child's general health and health-related quality of life as proxy's who are not blinded for the study group their child is in. This might bias the amount of HRQoL they report. Blinding parents was impossible because of the visual aspects of the intervention and the involvement of parents during the intervention. In a review Hack [21] warned that proxy HRQoL measurements can be influenced by parent's cultural, social and educational background and their specific experience with children. Mothers and fathers who completed the questionnaire in the NIDCAP intervention group in the second RCT were younger but the parents' educational level was comparable in the two groups. The response rate in this study was good and the sample seemed representative of the typical population of preterm infants with a gestational age < 32 weeks admitted to a Dutch NICU.

Most children received an optimal score of 100 on the TAPQoL scales. A recent study on the validity and reliability of the TAPQoL [17] warns that this 'ceiling effect' may limit the use of the TAPQoL to measure change. In the current study HRQoL scores were divided into three groups to try to divide scores more evenly.

Previous studies [10-13] have shown that very preterm born infants have less optimal HRQoL scores on some scales, compared to a reference group from the normal population. A study by Eiser [10] only found a difference between preterm and term infants on social HQoL but found no differences in the physical or emotional HQoL as reported by parents. A recent study on the HRQoL of Dutch preterm infants compared with term infants, using the TAPQoL at 1 year, showed significant lower HRQoL scores on the stomach, lungs and eating problems scales [12]. However, on other domains HRQoL scores of the preterm infants often scored optimal and were comparable to term infants. The stomach, lungs and eating problems scales seem to represent typical problems that preterm infants encounter. Basic DC and NIDCAP did not significantly improve HRQoL on these scales.

Conclusion

These two consecutive randomized controlled trials showed that neither a basic form of Developmental Care nor the more individualized NIDCAP intervention improved health-related quality of life of very preterm infants at 1 year of age.

Acknowledgements

We are grateful to the parents for taking the time and effort to fill in the questionnaires. We would also like to thank the medical and nursing staff at the Leiden University Medical Center and the Juliana Children's Hospital for their involvement in this study and ZONMW (grant 2100.0072) and the Health Care Efficiency Research Fund LUMC for funding this study.

References

1. Hansen,B.M. & Greisen,G. Is improved survival of very-low-birthweight infants in the 1980s and 1990s associated with increasing intellectual deficit in surviving children? *Dev. Med. Child Neurol.* **46**, 812-815 (2004).

2. Veen,S. *et al.* Impairments, disabilities, and handicaps of very preterm and very-low-birthweight infants at five years of age. The Collaborative Project on Preterm and Small for Gestational Age Infants (POPS) in The Netherlands. *Lancet* **338**, 33-36 (1991).

3. Als,H. Developmental Interventions in the Neonatal Intensive Care Nursery. Goldson,E. (ed.), pp. 18-85 (Oxford University Press, New York,1999).

4. Als,H. Towards a synactive theory of development: Promise for the assessment of infant individuality. *Infant Mental Health Journal* **3**, 229-243 (1982).

5. Als,H. & Gilkerson,L. The role of relationship-based developmentally supportive newborn intensive care in strengthening outcome of preterm infants. *Semin. Perinatol.* **21**, 178-189 (1997).

6. Symington,A. & Pinelli,J. Developmental care for promoting development and preventing morbidity in preterm infants. *Cochrane. Database. Syst. Rev.* CD001814 (2006).

7. Donohue,P.K. Health-related quality of life of preterm children and their caregivers. *Ment. Retard. Dev. Disabil. Res. Rev.* **8**, 293-297 (2002).

8. Verrips,E.G. *et al.* Measuring health-related quality of life in a child population. *Eur. J. Public Health* **9**, 188-193 (1999).

9. Vogels,T. *et al.* Measuring health-related quality of life in children: the development of the TACQOL parent form. *Qual. Life Res.* 7, 457-465 (1998).

10. Eiser,C., Eiser,J.R., Mayhew,A.G. & Gibson,A.T. Parenting the premature infant: balancing vulnerability and quality of life. *J. Child Psychol. Psychiatry* **46**, 1169-1177 (2005).

11. Klassen,A.F. *et al.* Health status and health-related quality of life in a population-based sample of neonatal intensive care unit graduates. *Pediatrics* **113**, 594-600 (2004).

12. Stoelhorst,G.M. Development, Quality of Life and Behavior at 2 Years of Age in Very Preterm Infants. Doctoral dissertation. Leiden University Medical Centre, Leiden (2003).

13. Theunissen,N.C. *et al.* Quality of life in preschool children born preterm. *Dev. Med. Child Neurol.* **43**, 460-465 (2001).

14. Fekkes,M. *et al.* Development and psychometric evaluation of the TAPQOL: a health-related quality of life instrument for 1-5-year-old children. *Qual. Life Res.* **9**, 961-972 (2000).

15. The International Neonatal Network. The CRIB (clinical risk index for babies) score: a tool for assessing initial neonatal risk and comparing performance of neonatal intensive care units. *Lancet* **342**, 193-198 (1993).

16. Fekkes,M., Bruil,J. & Vogels,T. TAPQOL manual. Leiden Center for Child Health and Pediatrics LUMC-TNO, Leiden (2004).

17. Bunge,E.M. *et al.* Reliability and validity of health status measurement by the TAPQOL. *Arch. Dis. Child* **90**, 351-358 (2005).

18. Brooks-Gunn,J. *et al.* Early intervention in low-birth-weight premature infants. Results through age 5 years from the Infant Health and Development Program. *JAMA* **272**, 1257-1262 (1994).

19. McCarton,C.M. *et al.* Results at age 8 years of early intervention for low-birth-weight premature infants. The Infant Health and Development Program. *JAMA* **277**, 126-132 (1997).

20. The Infant Health and Development Program. Enhancing the outcomes of low-birth-weight, premature infants. A multisite, randomized trial. *JAMA* **263**, 3035-3042 (1990).

21. Hack,M. Consideration of the use of health status, functional outcome, and quality-of-life to monitor neonatal intensive care practice. *Pediatrics* **103**, 319-328 (1999).

CHAPTER 4

Very preterm infant's behavior at 1 and 2 years of age and parental stress following basic Developmental Care

ylvia M. van der Pal
eleste M. Maguire
anet Bruil
askia le Cessie
aul van Zwieten
ylvia Veen
an Maarten Wit
rans J. Walther

Abstract

Objectives

To explore the effects of basic Developmental Care (DC) on the behavior of very preterm infants and parental stress at 1 and 2 years of corrected age.

Methods

Randomized Controlled Trial comparing basic DC (standardized nests and incubator covers) and controls (standard care). Parents of infants born < 32 weeks of gestation completed questionnaires measuring child behavior and parental stress at 1 year (n=139) and 2 years (n=133) of the child's age. Parental stress was measured using the Nijmegen Parenting Stress Index and child behavior was measured using the Infant-Toddler Social and Emotional Assessment and the Child Behavior Checklist 2-3.

Results

At 1 year of age children in the basic DC group had significantly higher behavior scores on the total competence domain (p=0.009) and the competence subscale mastery motivation (p=0.002), meaning that the infants showed more curiosity, persistence, obedience and enjoyment with small accomplishments. No significant effects were found on problem behavior or parenting stress.

Conclusion

Introducing a basic form of developmental care in the neonatal intensive care unit has a positive influence on the child's competence behavior at 1 year of age.

Introduction

Preterm infants show increased problem behavior compared to infants born at term. A meta-analysis [1] showed more externalizing and internalizing problem behavior in preterm infants in 13 out of 16 studies (81%) and more attention deficit hyperactivity disorder symptom behavior in 10 out of 15 studies (67%). In addition, parents of preterm infants report more stress [2,3] and experience more maladaptation and need for support during the first year after delivery [4] than parents of infants born at term. Holditch-Davis and colleagues [5] found that mothers of high-risk preterm infants experienced at least one of three symptoms of post-traumatic stress disorder (re-experiencing, avoidance and increased arousal), which might relate to their overall stress levels.

Parental or post-traumatic stress and infant behavior problems seem interrelated. In a study by Miceli and colleagues [6], the development and problem behavior of very preterm born infants at 36 months were related to maternal stress and depression at 4 months. Furthermore, the intensity of posttraumatic stress reactions after the preterm birth of parents of preterm infants correlates with the risk of the child developing sleeping and eating problems [7].

Advances in neonatology have decreased the mortality of infants born preterm [8,9]. To reduce morbidity and to support parents, neonatal caregiving in the neonatal intensive care unit (NICU) has shifted to a more individualized approach. In this context the Newborn Individualized Developmental Care and Assessment Program (NIDCAP) [10,11] was introduced in the 1980's. This program is based on individual observations of preterm infant behavior during caregiving that result in individual recommendations for caregiving.

A three-center NIDCAP intervention study in the United States showed positive outcomes on parental stress and infant behavior, such as improved self-regulation (motor and autonomic system) and less required facilitation on the Assessment of Preterm Infants' Behavior (APIB) at 2 weeks after the expected due date [12]. A study in Sweden found improved behavior after NIDCAP, as reported by parents at 3 years of age [13].

General developmental care based recommendations are reduced light, sound and activity levels in the NICU and the use of nests to support the infant's posture and incubator covers to decrease the light and sound level inside the incubator to provide an environment more comparable to the circumstances in the womb. The guidance by a NIDCAP-trained developmental specialist is intensive and costly. The implementation of the basic recommendations of developmental care is therefore often seen as a first step when implementing NIDCAP, before deciding to train staff members. In this context information needs to be provided about the effects of this basic form of developmental care.

The randomized controlled trial in the current study was designed to measure whether providing only basic developmental care (the use of standardized nests and covers) would have a positive long-term effect on very preterm infants' behavioral problems and their parents' stress at 1 and 2 years of age. We hypothesized that the protective characteristics of the nests and covers would allow the infants to rest and sleep more and become more alert and calm. The protective characteristics of the nests and covers might therefore improve the infant's self-regulation and behavior. Improved infant behavior and the sight of their infant being more comfortable in the nests and under the incubator covers was thought to reduce parental stress.

Methods

Subjects

Infants born with a gestational age (GA) below 32 weeks admitted to a NICU at two locations in the Netherlands (inclusion April 2000 – May 2002) were randomly assigned, by using sealed envelops, to a control or intervention group within 48 hours after birth.

Exclusion criteria were: infants of drug-addicted mothers and infants with congenital heart disease or other major birth anomalies. According to protocol, infants in both groups who were admitted for less then 5 days were excluded from follow-up because the duration of the basic DC intervention was hypothesized not to be long enough to measure effects. Based on the primary outcome of this study, the developmental tests at follow up, a sample size power calculation showed that 140 infants (70 controls, 70 intervention) were needed to show a significant difference with a power of 80%, based on the expected difference of half a standard deviation. We included more infants (a total of 192 infants) after parental informed consent was obtained, because of anticipated loss to follow up. The Medical Ethics Committees of both locations approved this study.

Basic Developmental Care Intervention

The basic developmental care (DC) intervention consisted of the reduction of light and sound inside the incubator through the use of standardized incubator covers. Standardized nests were used to support motor development and physiological stability by positioning the infant in ways that encourage flexion and containment. The control group received standard care prior to the beginning of this study when no incubator covers or forms of nesting were used. All infants were cared for in the same unit with the same light, sound and activity levels. Therefore, the only difference between the groups was the use of standardized incubator covers and nests. The nurses could not be blinded because of the visual aspects of the intervention. They received a clinical lesson about the use of the standardized materials.

Outcome Measures

All ages mentioned hereafter are corrected for prematurity (age corrected for gestational age at birth, thus time interval from term date). At 1 and 2 years of age the children were seen for follow-up by the neonatologist and parents were asked to complete a set of questionnaires.

Parent and child characteristics:

Demographic variables were obtained from the questionnaires and included parental age, educational level and country of birth (the Netherlands/other).

Infant characteristics at birth were obtained from the medical records and included gender, gestational age, birth weight and the Clinical Risk Index for Babies (CRIB) score. The CRIB score [14] assesses initial neonatal risk by scoring birth weight, gestational age, congenital malformation, maximal base excess in the first 12 hours and minimum and maximal oxygen requirements in the first 12 hours after birth.

Child behavior:
At 1 year of the infant's age, parents completed a Dutch translation of the Infant-Toddler Social and Emotional Assessment (ITSEA) [15]. This questionnaire was translated into Dutch and some items were deleted from the original questionnaire because of the young age of the infants. The following subscales were excluded from the original ITSEA: peer aggression, general anxiety (i.e. "worries about own body"), prosocial peer relations and the maladaptive scale. The modified questionnaire consisted of 15 behavior subscales, divided over 5 main factor domains: externalizing (activity/impulsivity and aggression/defiance), internalizing (depression/withdrawal, separation distress and inhibition to novelty), dysregulation (sleep problems, negative emotionality, eating problems, sensory sensitivity), competence (compliance, attention, imitation/play, mastery motivation, empathy) and social relatedness.

Other than the above described deleted subscales, zero to three items were removed from the remaining subscales in each domain. The modified questionnaire used in this study consisted of 107 items with answers on a 3 point Likert scale (0=not true/rarely, 1=somewhat true/sometimes, 2=very true/often). In a previous study the original questionnaire was validated [15]. In the current study alpha's ranged from 0.78 to 0.87 for all domains of the Dutch translated questionnaire, which is comparable to the Cronbach alpha's, ranging from 0.80 to 0.90 (and alpha of 0.56 for social relatedness), found for the domains of the original ITSEA [15]. The mean domain scores ranged from 0 to 2 and a higher score represented more problem or competence behavior.

At 2 years of age parents received the Child Behavior Checklist 2-3 yrs. (CBCL 2-3) [16]. The CBCL 2-3 includes 100 problem behavior items divided into 5 domains; total internalizing (anxiety/depressed and withdrawn), sleep problems, somatic problems, total externalizing (aggressive behavior and destructive behavior) and a total behavior score. Domain scores were calculated by adding the item scores within a scale. Mean test-retest reliability (0.87) of the CBCL was good [16] and in the current study Cronbach's alpha ranged from 0.57 (somatic problems) to 0.95. A higher total score (table 3 shows the range of total scores per scale) represented more problem or competence behavior.

Parenting Stress:

The Nijmegen Parenting Stress Index (NOSI) [17] is a Dutch version of the Parenting Stress Index (PSI) [18]. At 1 year parents were asked to complete the short version, the NOSIK. The NOSIK consists of 25 parental-stress-related statements (the items that performed best in the NOSI complete version) with answers on a 5 point Likert scale ranging from 1 (totally disagree) to 5 (totally agree). The NOSIK has a total parenting stress scale and a parent and child domain. The Cronbach's alpha score of the total scale of the short version, NOSIK, was good (α=0.95) [17] and this was also true in the present study (α=0.92).

The complete version, the NOSI, was given at two years of age and consists of 123 parental-stress-related statements with a total score and a child and parent domain. The parent domain contains the subscales: competence, parent role restriction, attachment, depression, health, isolation and spouse. The child domain contains the subscales: adaptability, mood, demandingness, distractibility/hyperactivity, reinforces parent and acceptability. Cronbach's alpha's of the domains (parent, child and total score) of the complete version, the NOSI, were good in earlier studies and ranged from 0.95 to 0.97 [17]. In this study the Cronbach's alpha reliability scores of the domains ranged from 0.93 to 0.95. The mean scale scores on the NOSI(K) ranged from 0 to 5 and a higher score represented more parenting stress.

Analysis

Mean scores were calculated for the domains and subscales of the ITSEA and NOSI(K). Mean scores were calculated when less than 30% of the items within a domain or subscale were missing. The CBCL domain scores represented a sum of all items belonging to the domains.

For statistical analysis SPSS 11.0 for Windows was used. Child and parent characteristics were compared with the Chi-square test, the Chi-square test for trend, the two-sample t-test or the non-parametric Mann-Whitney test, where appropriate.

Mean and total scale scores between groups were compared using a covariate analysis in which the infant and parent characteristics (parental age, educational level and country of birth (the Netherlands/other) and the infant's gender, gestational age, birth weight and CRIB score) and the completion day (the number of days between the infant's age of 1 and 2 years, corrected for prematurity, and the date when the parents completed the questionnaire) were included as covariates for a more precise estimation of the difference between the intervention and control groups and to correct for possible confounders. Because of multiple testing a p-value of below 0.01 was chosen as significance level.

The percentages of infants scoring high (> 95/90th percentile, compared to the reference groups) on problem behavior or parental stress, were reported and compared between both groups using a Chi square test. The CBCL reference group consisted of the scores of Dutch girls from a study by Koot [19] and the NOSI reference group was derived from the manual (scores of non-clinical Dutch mothers) [17]. The reference group of the ITSEA of 12-17 month old boys and girls in the USA as described in a study by Carte and collegues [15] was not used because a modified version of the ITSEA was used in the current study.

Results

Subjects

Figure 1 shows the loss to follow-up. The loss to follow-up in this figure also included infants transferred within 5 days of admission. One hundred and ninety two infants were included in this study (Figure 1). At 1 year, 139 questionnaires were returned of 146 sets of parents who received the questionnaire (return rate: 95% of received questionnaires and 83% of all included infants minus infant deaths).

At 2 years 133 questionnaires were returned (Figure 1) of the 142 sets of parents that received the questionnaire (return rates: 94% and 80%). At 2 years 1 set of parents in the control group and 6 sets of parents in the DC group forgot to fill in the CBCL behavior questionnaire on the last pages of the set of questionnaires.

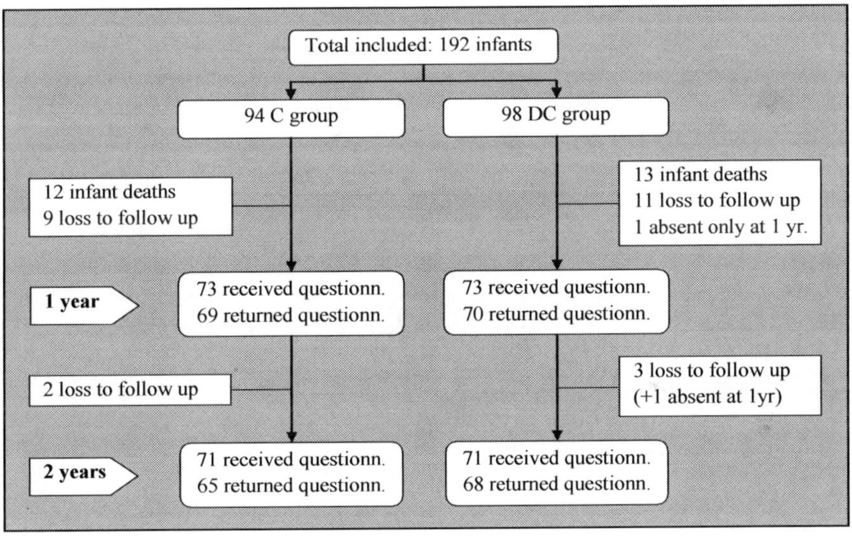

Figure 1. Loss to follow up and returned questionnaires.

The infant and parent characteristics were comparable between both groups within the returned questionnaires (Table 1), with the exception of the corrected age of the infant when completing the questionnaire at 2 years (p=.008). This variable was one of the covariates in the covariance analysis of the questionnaires.

Infant and parent characteristics		DC n(%) or mean(sd) N= 70	Control n(%) or mean(sd) N= 69	Difference p-value^
Gender (male)		37 (53%)	46 (67%)	.10
Gestational age at infant's birth (weeks)		29.5 (1.6)	29.1 (2.0)	.22
Birth weight (grams)		1249 (341)	1237 (324)	.84
CRIB score 14		3.2 (3.0)	3.7 (3.0)	.37
Duration of admission in intervention hospitals (days; median/range)		36.5 (6;100)	35 (5;114)	.50 ▫
Maternal age at infant's birth (years)		30.2 (5.1)	30.5 (4.8)	.74
Maternal education level #	low	31 (44%)	22 (32%)	.25
	intermediate	23 (33%)	28 (41%)	
	high	16 (23%)	18 (27%)	
Country of birth mother (the Netherlands)		48 (69%)	53 (77%)	.28
Paternal age at birth infant (years)		33.1 (5.3)	33.8 (5.7)	.47
Paternal education level #	low	27 (39%)	16 (24%)	.12
	intermediate	25 (36%)	31 (46%)	
	high	17 (25%)	20 (30%)	
Country of birth father (the Netherlands)		52 (74%)	55 (80%)	.45
Completed by ...	mother	48 (70%)	48 (72%)	.81
	father	8 (12%)	9 (13%)	
	both	13 (19%)	10 (15%)	
Completing day after age 1 years (days; median/range)		15 (-12;95)	9.5 (-11;117)	.10 ▫
Completing day after age 2 years (days; median/range)		18 (-14;213)	9 (-13;112)	.008 * ▫

Table 1. Comparison of infant and parent characteristics of completed questionnaires at 1 year.

* p < .01

^ Two sample t-test / Chi square test (for trend)

\# Low = vocational education, intermediate = high school, high = college education/ university

▫ Non parametric Mann-Whitney test

There were no significant differences in gender, gestational age at birth and birth weight, within the infants whose parents did not receive or complete the questionnaire (non-responders: 1 year: controls N=25, basic DC N=28, 2 years: controls N=29, basic DC N=30, data not shown).

Behavior According to ITSEA and CBCL Parent Questionnaires

Table 2 shows that at 1 year of age (ITSEA) the mean scores of the total Competence domain were better in the DC group compared to the controls (difference (99%CI)= 0.15 (0.003;0.30), p=0.009). Within the subscales of the competence domain, children in the DC group had significantly better mastery motivation competence mean scores compared to the controls (difference (99%CI)= 0.20 (0.03;0.37), p=0.002), which indicates that children in the DC group showed more curiosity, persistence and enjoyment with small accomplishments. Although mean scores on problem behavior at 1 year tended to be higher in the DC group, indicating more problem behavior, this difference did not reach statistical significance.

ITSEA Domain scores (range 0-2)	DC N=70 (min n=67)	C N=69 (min n=67)	DC-C Difference #
Problem behavior	**Mean (sd)**	**Mean (sd)**	**Difference (99% CI) #**
Externalizing	.50 (.30)	.38 (.28)	.06 (-.06;.19)
Internalizing	.52 (.26)	.44 (.26)	.05 (-.07;.17)
Dysregulation	.45 (.26)	.39 (.21)	.005 (-.10;.11)
Competence behavior	**Mean (sd)**	**Mean (sd)**	**Diff (99% CI) #**
Competence	1.16 (.29)	1.03 (.33)	.15 (.003;.30)*
Mastery Motivation ~	1.57 (.32)	1.41 (.37)	.20 (.03;.37)*
Social Relatedness	1.64 (.27)	1.60 (.29)	.08 (-.06;.21)

Table 2. Comparison DC and C on infant behavior at 1 year (ITSEA) of corrected age.

* p < .01

\# Covariance analysis; difference (99% CI), corrected for the completion day after the age of 1 year, infant gender, gestational age, birth weight, CRIB and the age, educational level and country of birth of parents. Min N DC=62, C=65

~ Subscale of competence domain of ITSEA

. For all ITSEA domains: higher mean score represents more behavior problems/competence

At 2 years of age no significant differences were found between the two groups on child behavior problems using the CBCL 2-3 (Table 3). The percentages of infants scoring non-optimal on problem behavior also did not differ between the two groups.

CBCL 2 years Problem behavior	DC N=62	C N=64	DC-C Difference #	DC % non optimal	C % non optimal
Scale scores (range)	**Mean(sd)**	**Mean(sd)**	**Diff (99% CI) #**	**%(n) ≥95 perc.**	**%(n) ≥95 perc.**
Sleep Problems (0-14)	2.4 (2.3)	2.8 (2.9)	**-.38 (-1.62;.86)**	8.1 % (5)	7.8 % (5)
Somatic Problems (0-28)	2.7 (2.4)	3.1 (2.5)	**-.50 (-1.75;.76)**	6.5 % (4)	10.9 % (7)
				%(n) ≥90 perc.	**%(n) ≥90 perc.**
Internalizing (0-50)	5.1 (4.7)	5.7 (4.7)	**-.40 (-2.73;1.93)**	8.1 % (5)	10.9 % (7)
Externalizing (0-52)	10.8 (7.3)	11.0 (8.1)	**.20 (-3.41; 3.80)**	11.3 % (7)	12.5 % (8)
Total Behavior (0-198)	27.2 (18.1)	29.0 (20.2)	**-1.12 (-10.4;8.1)**	9.7 % (6)	14.1 % (9)

Table 3. Comparison DC and C on infant behavior at 2 years (CBCL) of corrected age.

\# Covariance analysis; difference (99% CI), corrected for the completion day after the age of 2 years, infant gender, gestational age, birth weight, CRIB and the age, educational level and country of birth of parents. Min N DC=57, C=59

For all CBCL scales: higher mean score represents more problem behavior

Parenting Stress

At 1 and 2 years of age no significant differences were found between the two groups on parenting stress (Table 4). Although parental stress at 2 years tended to be higher in the DC group, this difference was not statistically significant and the percentages of parents scoring non-optimal did not differ between the two groups.

	DC Mean(sd)	C Mean(sd)	DC-C Difference #	DC % non optimal	C % non optimal
NOSIK (short version) 1 year	**N=70**	**N=69**	**diff.(99%CI) #**	**%(n) ≥90 perc.**	**%(n) ≥90 perc.**
Total score Parent Domain	1.74 (.71)	1.70 (.67)	**.03 (-.29;.35)**		
Total score Child Domain	1.95 (.77)	1.78 (.76)	**.11 (-.21;.43)**		
Total Stress score	1.86 (.70)	1.75 (.68)	**.08 (-.23;.38)**	9 % (6)	3 % (2)
NOSI 2 years	**N=67**	**N=65**	**diff.(99%CI) #**	**%(n) ≥90 perc.**	**%(n) ≥90 perc.**
Total score Parent Domain	2.06 (.67)	1.85 (.64)	**.22 (-.13;.56)**	16 % (11)	15 % (10)
Total score Child Domain	2.08 (.52)	1.91 (.52)	**.16 (-.10;.42)**	12 % (8)	8 % (5)
Total Stress score	2.07 (.55)	1.89 (.53)	**.19 (-.09;.46)**	16 % (11)	8 % (5)

Table 4. Comparison DC and C on parenting stress at 1 year (NOSIK, short version) and 2 years (NOSI) of corrected age

\# Covariance analysis; difference (99% CI), corrected for the completion day after the age of 1 or 2 years, infant gender, gestational age, birth weight, CRIB and the age, educational level and country of birth of parents. Min N 1yr: DC=64, C=66, 2 yrs: DC=62, C=59

For all NOSI(K) scales: higher mean score represents more parental stress (range 0-5)

Discussion

This randomized controlled trial demonstrated that very preterm infants who received basic elements of developmental care (standardized nests and incubator covers) showed more competence behavior at 1 year of age, especially regarding mastery motivation. Parents of children that received basic Developmental Care reported that their child showed more curiosity, persistence and enjoyment with small accomplishments and that they were more often well-behaved and obedient. While competence behavior at 1 year was improved in the basic DC group, parents also tended to report more problem behavior at 1 year, but this small difference had disappeared by 2 years of age. At 2 years of age we used the CBCL 2-3 because this questionnaire is often used in the Netherlands and in other intervention studies. This questionnaire only included problem behavior items and no competence behavior items and therefore it was not possible to test the continuation of improved competence behavior at 2 years of age.

Although parents in the DC group reported that their child showed more competence behavior, there were no significant differences between the groups in parental stress. The improved competence behavior found in this study therefore does not seem to be related to a decrease in parental stress as expected in the context of the correlation of parental stress and child behavior found in previous studies [6,7].

The children and parents in this study had problem behavior and stress scores comparable to reference groups from the normal population. A meta-analysis showed that previous studies found more behavior problem in preterm infants [1]. Most behavioral impairment was found in studies with infants < 30 weeks of gestation [1], while the infants included in this study were < 32 weeks of gestation. A recent study with Dutch preterm infants < 32 weeks also showed that the prevalence of behavior problems was comparable to term infants using the CBCL 2-3 at 2 years of age [20].

Previous studies on the effect of the complete NIDCAP intervention with individual observations and guidance found positive effects on infant behavior and parental stress. These effects were mainly found around the expected due date, such as improved behavior on the Assessment of Preterm Infant Behavior (APIB) test at 2 weeks of age, corrected for prematurity [12,21,22], improved emotional regulation and motor quality on the BSID II Behavior Rating Scale at 9 months of corrected age [21] and improved parental stress at 2 weeks corrected age, using the Parenting Stress Index [12]. A Swedish study reported improved child behavior on the Höök-Cederblad Child Behaviour Interview and improved child communication on the Early Relational Assessment at 3 years of age [13]. At 5 years of age, a higher, however non-significant, percentage of survival without attention deficits was found in the NIDCAP group [23]. The authors of the Swedish study call for caution in interpreting their results because of a small sample size. Kaaresen and colleagues [24] studied the effects of a modified version of the Mother-Infant Transaction Program with 8 sessions during admission and 4 home visits after discharge. They found a decrease on the total parental stress domain and on both the parent and child domains of the Parenting Stress Index questionnaire at 6 and 12 months of corrected age.

In the current study, no effects were found of a basic form of developmental care on parental stress or problem behavior during follow-up at 1 and 2 years of age. A more individualized approach, such as the individual behavior observation and recommendations and the guidance of parents of the complete NIDCAP intervention, might decrease parental stress and decrease problem behavior of the infants. Further research that explores the effects of a more individualized form of Developmental Care, such as the NIDCAP, on child behavior and parental stress in the first year after intervention is needed.

Two intervention studies regarding the Infant Health and Development Program, (IHDP; home visits, child development center services and parent group meetings until 3 years of age in the USA) and the Avon Premature Infant Project (APIP; two interventions consisting of weekly home visits up to 2 years of age, a developmental education program and a social support intervention in the UK) found less problem behavior on the CBCL after the intervention ended at respectively 3 and 2 years of age but no significant differences were found at follow up at 5 years [25,26] and 8 years of age [27]. An intervention with weekly home visits for 8 weeks, resulted in improved competence behavior, such as better problem solving and activity, cooperation, general emotional tone and vocalization at 7 months of age [28]. These studies on the effect of interventions with preterm infants show effects on child competence behavior but not on behavior problems at follow up. The current study also found no effects on problem behavior but did find an effect on competence behavior. There seems to exist an opportunity for interventions to positively influence competence behavior, which is also an important part of the behavioral spectrum. Future research on the effect of interventions at the NICU should, besides exploring effects on problem behavior, also focus on the child's competence behavior.

In conclusion, this study shows that basic developmental care (the use of standardized nests and covers) during the admission of very preterm infants does not have a significant effect on the child's problem behavior and parental stress at 1 and 2 years of age. However, problem behavior and parental stress scores in the current study did not seem to differ much from term reference groups. There appeared to be a window of opportunity to improve the child's competence behavior and this study found a significant effect of the basic elements of developmental care on competence (mastery motivation) behavior at 1 year of age. The effects of basic DC on the infant's growth and development will be described elsewhere and are also of importance before recommendations for implementation can be given. This study shows that basic developmental care has a positive effect on infant competence behavior at 1 year and this form of developmental care seems easy to implement.

Acknowledgements

We are grateful to the parents for taking the time and effort to complete the questionnaires. We would also like to thank the medical and nursing staff at the Leiden University Medical Center and the Juliana Children's Hospital for their involvement in carrying out this study and ZONMW (grant 2100.0072) and the Health Care Efficiency Research Fund LUMC for funding this study.

References

1. Bhutta,A.T., Cleves,M.A., Casey,P.H., Cradock,M.M. & Anand,K.J. Cognitive and behavioral outcomes of school-aged children who were born preterm: a meta-analysis. *JAMA* **288**, 728-737 (2002).

2. Lau,R. & Morse,C.A. Stress experiences of parents with premature infants in a special care nursery. *Stress and Health* **19**, 69-78 (2003).

3. Singer,L.T. *et al.* Maternal psychological distress and parenting stress after the birth of a very low-birth-weight infant. *JAMA* **281**, 799-805 (1999).

4. Rautava,P., Lehtonen,L., Helenius,H. & Sillanpaa,M. Effect of newborn hospitalization on family and child behavior: a 12-year follow-up study. *Pediatrics* **111**, 277-283 (2003).

5. Holditch-Davis,D., Bartlett,T.R., Blickman,A.L. & Miles,M.S. Posttraumatic stress symptoms in mothers of premature infants. *J. Obstet. Gynecol. Neonatal Nurs.* **32**, 161-171 (2003).

6. Miceli,P.J. *et al.* Brief report: birth status, medical complications, and social environment: individual differences in development of preterm, very low birth weight infants. *J. Pediatr. Psychol.* **25**, 353-358 (2000).

7. Pierrehumbert,B., Nicole,A., Muller-Nix,C., Forcada-Guex,M. & Ansermet,F. Parental post-traumatic reactions after premature birth: implications for sleeping and eating problems in the infant. *Arch. Dis. Child Fetal Neonatal Ed* **88**, F400-F404 (2003).

8. Hansen,B.M. & Greisen,G. Is improved survival of very-low-birthweight infants in the 1980s and 1990s associated with increasing intellectual deficit in surviving children? *Dev. Med. Child Neurol.* **46**, 812-815 (2004).

9. Veen,S. *et al.* Impairments, disabilities, and handicaps of very preterm and very-low-birthweight infants at five years of age. The Collaborative Project on Preterm and Small for Gestational Age Infants (POPS) in The Netherlands. *Lancet* **338**, 33-36 (1991).

10. Als,H. Developmental Interventions in the Neonatal Intensive Care Nursery. Goldson,E. (ed.), pp. 18-85 (Oxford University Press, New York,1999).

11. Als,H. & Gilkerson,L. The role of relationship-based developmentally supportive newborn intensive care in strengthening outcome of preterm infants. *Semin. Perinatol.* **21**, 178-189 (1997).

12. Als,H. *et al.* A three-center, randomized, controlled trial of individualized developmental care for very low birth weight preterm infants: medical, neurodevelopmental, parenting, and caregiving effects. *J. Dev. Behav. Pediatr.* **24**, 399-408 (2003).

13. Kleberg,A., Westrup,B. & Stjernqvist,K. Developmental outcome, child behaviour and mother-child interaction at 3 years of age following Newborn Individualized Developmental Care and Intervention Program (NIDCAP) intervention. *Early Hum. Dev.* **60**, 123-135 (2000).

14. The International Neonatal Network. The CRIB (clinical risk index for babies) score: a tool for assessing initial neonatal risk and comparing performance of neonatal intensive care units. *Lancet* **342**, 193-198 (1993).

15. Carter,A.S., Briggs-Gowan,M.J., Jones,S.M. & Little,T.D. The Infant-Toddler Social and Emotional Assessment (ITSEA): factor structure, reliability, and validity. *J. Abnorm. Child Psychol.* **31**, 495-514 (2003).

16. Achenbach,T.M., Edelbrock,C. & Howell,C.T. Empirically based assessment of the behavioral/emotional problems of 2- and 3- year-old children. *J. Abnorm. Child Psychol.* **15**, 629-650 (1987).

17. de Brock,A.J.L.L., Vermulst,A.A., Gerris,J.R.M. & Abidin,R.R. NOSI - Nijmeegse Ouderlijke Stress Index, Handleiding experimentele versie [NOSI- Nijmegen Parenting Stress Index, Manual experimental version]. Swets en Zeitlinger, Lisse (1992).

18. Abidin,R.R. Parenting Stress Index. Pediatric Psychology Press, Charlottesville (1983).

19. Koot,J.M. Problem Behavior in Dutch Preschoolers. Doctoral dissertation. Erasmus University Rotterdam, Rotterdam (1993).

20. Stoelhorst,G.M. *et al.* Behaviour at 2 years of age in very preterm infants (gestational age < 32 weeks). *Acta Paediatr.* **92**, 595-601 (2003).

21. Als,H. *et al.* Early experience alters brain function and structure. *Pediatrics* **113**, 846-857 (2004).

22. Buehler,D.M., Als,H., Duffy,F.H., McAnulty,G.B. & Liederman,J. Effectiveness of individualized developmental care for low-risk preterm

infants: behavioral and electrophysiologic evidence. *Pediatrics* **96**, 923-932 (1995).

23. Westrup,B., Bohm,B., Lagercrantz,H. & Stjernqvist,K. Preschool outcome in children born very prematurely and cared for according to the Newborn Individualized Developmental Care and Assessment Program (NIDCAP). *Acta Paediatr.* **93**, 498-507 (2004).

24. Kaaresen,P.I., Ronning,J.A., Ulvund,S.E. & Dahl,L.B. A randomized, controlled trial of the effectiveness of an early-intervention program in reducing parenting stress after preterm birth. *Pediatrics* **118**, e9-19 (2006).

25. Brooks-Gunn,J. *et al.* Early intervention in low-birth-weight premature infants. Results through age 5 years from the Infant Health and Development Program. *JAMA* **272**, 1257-1262 (1994).

26. Johnson,S., Ring,W., Anderson,P. & Marlow,N. Randomised trial of parental support for families with very preterm children: outcome at 5 years. *Arch. Dis. Child* **90**, 909-915 (2005).

27. McCarton,C.M. *et al.* Results at age 8 years of early intervention for low-birth-weight premature infants. The Infant Health and Development Program. *JAMA* **277**, 126-132 (1997).

28. Gardner,J.M., Walker,S.P., Powell,C.A. & Grantham-McGregor,S. A randomized controlled trial of a home-visiting intervention on cognition and behavior in term low birth weight infants. *J. Pediatr.* **143**, 634-639 (2003).

CHAPTER 5

Parental stress and child behavior and temperament in the first year after the Newborn Individualized Developmental Care and Assessment Program (NIDCAP)

LVIA M. VAN DER PAL
ELESTE M. MAGUIRE
SKIA LE CESSIE
LVIA VEEN
N MAARTEN WIT
RANS J. WALTHER
ANET BRUIL

CEPTED FOR PUBLICATION IN JOURNAL OF EARLY INTERVENTION

Abstract

A randomized controlled trial compared basic developmental care (nests and incubator covers) and the Newborn Individualized Developmental Care and Assessment Program (NIDCAP) intervention (behavior observations and guidance by a trained developmental specialist) to evaluate the effect of NIDCAP on parental stress and infant behavior and temperament during the preterm infant's first year of life (n=128). The NIDCAP group tended to show more social relatedness behavior (p=0.011) at 1 year, especially when admitted > 1.5 months at the NICU where the intervention took place (n=44; p=0.006). Parents in the NIDCAP group reported positive experiences and effects on the well-being of their infant during admission. No effects were found on temperament, problem behavior or parental stress. Implications for NIDCAP implementation are discussed.

Introduction

The occurrence of a preterm birth affects both the infant and the family. Parents of preterm infants report more stress [1,2] and experience more maladaptation and need for support during the first year after delivery [3] than parents of infants born at term. Mothers of preterm infants showed symptoms of post-traumatic stress syndrome in a study by Holditch-Davis and colleagues [4]. Preterm infants showed more externalizing and internalizing behavior problems in a meta-analysis in 13 out of 16 studies (81%) and more attention deficit hyperactivity disorder symptom behavior in 10 out of 15 studies (67%) [5]. The (posttraumatic) stress of parents of very preterm infants furthermore correlated with more problem behavior of their children at 36 months [6] and increased sleeping and eating problems as reported by parents [7].

Focus in neonatal caregiving has shifted to a more individualized approach with more emphasis on the family and in this context the Newborn Individualized Developmental Care and Assessment Program (NIDCAP) [8] was introduced in the 1980's. This program is based on the synactive theory of development [9] where the infant's individual behavior is observed along four channels of communication: autonomic system (skin colour, respiration etc.), motor system (posture, tone and movements), state organization system (type and range of states available to the infant from sleep to aroused and state transition) and attention and interaction system (the infant's ability to come to an alert, attentive state and to utilize this state to handle stimuli from the environment), by a NIDCAP trained developmental specialist. The infant's efforts at self-regulation and interaction are observed through approach and avoidance behaviors [9,10]. A narrative of the observation is written and individual recommendations to modify the infant's environment and caregiving, based on the observation, are discussed with parents and other caregivers and parents are supported in becoming more actively involved in the caregiving process [8,11]. An example of a recommendation based on the infant's behavior is the timing of pauses during caregiving, based on the infant's individual behavioral cues. An example of involving parents in caregiving is giving them recommendations how to comfort their child during the caregiving by the nurse.

The results of NIDCAP intervention studies in the United States and Sweden show positive outcomes [12-19]. A randomized controlled trial in three centers in the United States found less parental stress at 2 weeks after the expected date of confinement in a NIDCAP intervention group [13]. A Swedish study found a positive impact of NIDCAP on behavior at preschool age [19]. A recent review on the effects of various forms of Developmental Care [20] concluded that although limited benefits and no major harmful effects were found, the significant effects were mainly based on studies with small sample sizes and that several of these findings were not supported in other settings.

This study explores the effect of the individualized and family centered NIDCAP program on infant temperament at 9 months and infant behavior and parental stress at 1 year of the infant's corrected age, in comparison with a basic form of developmental care. We expected that the NIDCAP intervention would have more effect when the duration of the intervention was longer. In this context, the effect of the NIDCAP was also studied within a subgroup of infants who were admitted for more than 1.5 months at the NICU where the study took place.

Methods

NIDCAP intervention

A randomized controlled trial was conducted to explore the effect of individual care plans and guidance through the use of the NIDCAP (Newborn Individualized Developmental Care and Assessment Program) behavioral and observation tool [8,11], compared to a basic form of developmental care (nests and incubator covers). The intervention consisted of NIDCAP observations of the infant before, during and after the caregiving [8] every 7 to 10 days by a NIDCAP trained developmental specialist. The trained developmental specialist wrote reports and discussed individual recommendations with parents and other caregivers and supported them in giving care to the infant. The first observation was done within 48 hours after birth. A nursing team that had received additional clinical lessons in the NIDCAP approach was assigned to the infants in the NIDCAP intervention group. The control group received the basic elements of DC and was given nests to support flexed positioning and incubator covers to shield the infants from light and sound stimuli. These basic elements of developmental care are often seen as a first step for hospitals before they decide to train personnel, which costs more time and money. This study wanted to explore the additional value of the individualized approach of the NIDCAP observations and guidance.

Subjects

Infants born from July 2002 to August 2004 with a gestational age below 32 weeks in a NICU at two locations in the Netherlands were randomly assigned (sealed envelops with cards) to a control or NIDCAP group within 48 hours after birth. Exclusion criteria were: infants of drug-addicted mothers and infants with congenital heart disease or other major birth anomalies. According to protocol, infants in both the NIDCAP and basic DC control group who were admitted for less then 5 days were excluded from follow-up analysis because the duration of the NIDCAP intervention was hypothesized not to be long enough to measure any effect. A sample size power calculation showed that 140 infants (70 control and 70 intervention) were needed to show a significant difference with a power of 80%, based on the expected difference of half a standard deviation on the primary outcome (Bayley Scales of Infant Development, standard deviation of 15). In total 168 infants were included after parental informed consent was obtained. The Medical Ethics Committees of both locations approved this study.

Measures

All ages mentioned hereafter are corrected for prematurity. At 9 months of age the Infant Behavior Questionnaire Revised (IBQ-R) [21] was sent to the home address of parents to measure infant temperament. At the infant's age of 1 year, parents were given a modified version of the Infant-Toddler Social and Emotional Assessment (ITSEA) [22] to measure infant behavior and the Nijmegen Parenting Stress Index short version (NOSIK) [23], which measures parenting stress, at the follow-up clinic. Parents were asked to give their general opinion regarding the positive or negative effects that the control or intervention care had on their infant in an open question on the final page of the questionnaires given at 1 year.

Parent and child characteristics:

Demographic variables included parental age, educational level and country of birth (the Netherlands/other). Infant characteristics at birth included gender, gestational age, birth weight and the Clinical Risk Index for Babies (CRIB) score. The CRIB score [24] assesses initial neonatal risk by scoring birth weight, gestational age, congenital malformation, maximal base excess in the first 12 hours and minimum and maximal oxygen requirements in the first 12 hours after birth.

Infant temperament (IBQ-R) at 9 months:

At 9 months of their infant's age, parents completed the Infant Behavior Questionnaire Revised (IBQ-R) [21]. This questionnaire contains 191 behavior items which can be rated on a 7 point Likert scale (1=not present, 7=always present) with an extra "does not apply" answer possibility which received no numerical score when calculating mean scores for the scales. The items measured 14 behavior scales being: distress to limitations, fear, sadness, rate recovery from distress, activity level, smiling and laughter, high intensity pleasure, perceptual sensitivity, approach/positive anticipation, vocal reactivity, duration of orienting, low intensity pleasure, soothability and cuddliness. Cronbach's alpha for scale reliability (with infants 9-12 months) ranged from 0.71-0.87 [21] in a previous study. In the current study alpha's ranged from 0.74-0.89. The IBQ was translated forward/backwards into Dutch (translated from English into Dutch and then checked by having a native English speaker translate it back into English). The questionnaire and permission to use it were obtained from the author.

Infant behavior (modified ITSEA) at 1 year:

At 1 year of the infant's age parents completed a Dutch translation of the Infant-Toddler Social and Emotional Assessment (ITSEA) [22]. This questionnaire was translated into Dutch and some items were deleted from the original questionnaire because of the young age of the infants. The following subscales were excluded from the original ITSEA: peer aggression, general anxiety (i.e. "worries about own body"), prosocial peer relations and the maladaptive scale. The modified questionnaire consisted of 15 behavior subscales, divided over 5 main factor domains: externalizing (activity/impulsivity and aggression/defiance), internalizing (depression/withdrawal, separation distress and inhibition to novelty), dysregulation (sleep problems, negative emotionality, eating problems, sensory sensitivity), competence (compliance, attention, imitation/play, mastery motivation, empathy) and social relatedness.

Other than the above described deleted subscales, zero to three items were removed from the remaining subscales in each domain. The modified questionnaire used in this study consisted of 107 items with answers on a 3 point Likert scale (0=not true/rarely, 1=somewhat true/sometimes, 2=very true/often). In a previous study the original questionnaire was validated [22]. In the current study alpha's ranged from 0.80 to 0.86 (alpha of 0.80 for social relatedness) for domains of the Dutch translated questionnaire. This is comparable to the Cronbach alpha's, ranging from 0.88 to 0.94 (and an alpha of 0.56 for social relatedness), found for the domains of the original ITSEA [22], which suggests that the exclusion of items did not affect the reliability of the domains. The mean domain scores ranged from 0 to 2 and a higher score represented more problem or competence behavior.

Parenting Stress (NOSIK) at 1 year:
The Nijmegen Parenting Stress Index (NOSI) [23] is a Dutch version of the Parenting Stress Index (PSI) [25]. At 1 year parents were asked to complete the short version, the NOSIK. The NOSIK consists of 25 parental stress related statements (the items that performed best in the NOSI complete version) with answers on a 5 point Likert scale ranging from 1 (totally disagree) to 5 (totally agree). The NOSIK has a total parenting stress scale and a parent and a child domain. The Cronbach's alpha score of the total scale of the short version, NOSIK, was good (α=0.95) [23] and this was confirmed in the present study (α=0.94).

Analysis
For statistical analysis SPSS 11.0 for Windows was used. Average scale scores were calculated using the non-missing items, if the scale contained no more than 30% missing items. The infant and parent characteristics were

compared with the Chi-square test, the Chi-square test for trend, the two-sample t-test or the non-parametric Mann-Whitney test, where appropriate.

Mean scale scores of the two groups were compared using a covariate analysis in which the infant and parent characteristics and the completion day after the age of 1 year were included as covariates. This was done for a more precise estimation of the difference between the two groups and to correct for possible confounders. The effect of the NIDCAP intervention was also explored (covariance analysis) within a subgroup of infants who were admitted for > 45 days at the NICU where the study took place.

The percentages of parents scoring high (>90th percentile) on parental stress were reported and compared between both groups using a NOSIK reference group consisting of non-clinical Dutch mothers, derived from the manual [23]. Because of multiple testing a significance level of below 0.01 was chosen.

Results

Subjects

During the RCT 168 infants were included. At 9 months 146 parents received the IBQ questionnaire of which 134 (92%) were returned (Figure 1). The return rate of all 168 included children (minus 14 infant deaths) was 87%. At 1 year 144 parents received the questionnaire of which 128 (89%) were returned (Figure 1). The return rate of all 168 included children (minus 14 infant deaths) was 83%. The loss to follow-up as displayed in Figure 1 also included infants transferred within 5 days of admission.

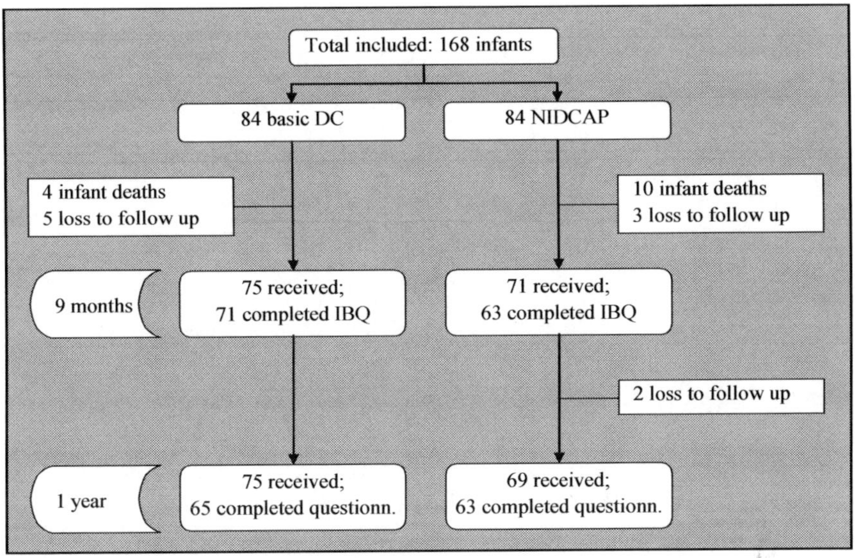

Figure 1. Loss to follow up and returned questionnaires.

The infant and parent characteristics of the parents who returned the questionnaire at 1 year were similar in both groups (Table 1), with the exception of maternal age (p=0.007), which was added as one of the covariates in the final covariance analysis. Mothers in NIDCAP intervention group were on average 2 years younger compared to mothers in the basic DC group and mothers in both groups were on average in their early thirties when completing the questionnaire.

		NIDCAP	Basic DC	Difference
		n(%) or mean(sd)	n(%) or mean(sd)	p-value ^
RCT (intervention: NIDCAP - control: basic DC)		N= 63	N= 65	
Completed by ...	mother	50 (79%)	57 (89%)	.32
	father	9 (14%)	5 (8%)	
	both	4 (6%)	2 (3%)	
Gender (male)		38 (60%)	33 (51%)	.28
Gestational age at birth (weeks)		29.6 (1.5)	29.2 (1.6)	.17
Birth Weight (grams)		1269 (318)	1244 (349)	.67
CRIB score 24		2.8 (2.8)	3.0 (3.1)	.70
Maternal age at infant's birth (yrs)		29.9 (5.1)	32.3 (4.9)	.007*
Maternal education level #	low	17 (27%)	12 (19%)	.31
	intermediate	24 (38%)	26 (41%)	
	high	22 (35%)	26 (41%)	
Country of birth mother (the Netherlands)		51 (81%)	58 (91%)	.12
Paternal age at infant's birth (yrs)		32.1 (5.8)	33.9 (5.5)	.08
Paternal education level #	low	12 (20%)	9 (15%)	.65
	intermediate	20 (34%)	32 (52%)	
	high	27 (46%)	21 (34%)	
Country of birth father (the Netherlands)		48 (77%)	50 (78%)	.92
Duration of admission in NICU where study took place (days)▫		38 (6;160)	36 (5;286)	.60
Completion after infant's age 9 months (days)▫		6 (-35;163)	7 (-12;140)	.66
Completion after infant's age 1 yrs (days)▫		9.5 (-35;119)	15 (-42;101)	.40

Table 1. Comparison of infant and parent characteristics of completed questionnaires at 1 year.

* p < .01

^ T-test / Chi-square test (for trend)

~ Low = vocational education, intermediate = high school, high = college education/ university

▫ Non parametric Mann-Whitney test (median and range per group)

Within the group of included infants whose parents did not receive or complete the questionnaire at 1 year (because of death or loss to follow up and nonresponders), both groups (basic DC N=19, NIDCAP n=21) were comparable concerning their gender, gestational age at birth and birth weight (data not shown).

Infant temperament at 9 months

No significant differences were found on the subscales of the IBQ measuring infant temperament.

IBQ 9 months; 1(never) -7(often) ~	NIDCAP mean (sd)	Basic DC mean (sd)	NIDCAP-DC Difference (99% CI) #
Distress to limitations	3.45 (.93)	3.45 (1.05)	.02 (-.48;.53)
Fear	2.59 (.68)	2.47 (.87)	.06 (-.33;.44)
Sadness	3.29 (.99)	3.35 (1.02)	-.11 (-.64;.42)
Rate recovery from distress	5.44 (.87)	5.44 (.92)	.02 (-.43;.48)
Activity level	3.88 (.92)	4.15 (.85)	-.33 (-.78;.12)
Smiling and laughter	5.15 (.91)	5.25 (.74)	-.03 (-.45;.40)
High pleasure	5.99 (.64)	6.04 (.61)	.05 (-.27;.36)
Perceptual sensitivity	4.00 (1.28)	4.33 (1.37)	- .40 (-1.18;.38)
Approach	5.15 (.69)	5.09 (.69)	.19 (-.17;.55)
Vocal reactivity	4.71 (.82)	4.75 (.86)	-.02 (-.48;.43)
Duration of orienting	3.74 (.98)	3.47 (1.06)	.26 (-.29;.81)
Low pleasure	5.24 (.88)	5.48 (.80)	-.08 (-.54;.39)
Soothability	5.53 (.84)	5.51 (.74)	.03 (-.40;.46)
Cuddliness	5.42 (.87)	5.48 (.78)	-.07 (-.50;.37)

Table 2: Infant temperament at 6 months (IBQ)

~ Higher scores represent the child displaying more of the behavior as described

Covariance analysis; difference (99% CI), corrected for the completion day after the age of 9 months, infant gender, gestational age, birth weight, CRIB and the age, educational level and country of birth of parents. Minimal N covariance: NIDCAP=49, basic DC=45.

Infant behavior at 1 year

No significant differences were found on infant behavior at 1 year between both groups. Social relatedness behavior tended to be higher in the NIDCAP group, compared to the infants that received basic DC (p=0.011).

ITSEA 1 yr (range 0-2) Mean score on domain	NIDCAP mean (sd)	Basic DC mean (sd)	NIDCAP-DC Difference #
Problem behavior ~			**Diff (99% CI) #**
Externalizing	.53 (.32)	.43 (.28)	.07 (-.09;.22)
Internalizing	.52 (.25)	.47 (.23)	.07 (-.05;.20)
Dysregulation	.45 (.28)	.42 (.22)	.02 (-.11;.14)
Competences ~			
Competence	1.06 (.30)	1.04 (.31)	.03 (-.12;.18)
Social Relatedness	1.71 (.20)	1.63 (.25)	.11 (-.001;.23)*

Table 3. Comparison NIDCAP and basic DC on infant behavior (ITSEA) at 1 year of corrected age.

* p < .05

\# Covariance analysis; difference(99% CI), corrected for the completion day after the age of 1 year, infant gender, gestational age, birth weight, CRIB and the age, educational level and country of birth of parents. N covariance: NIDCAP=58, basic DC=61.

~ For all ITSEA total domains: higher mean score represents more problem / competence behavior

Parenting stress at 1 year

No significant differences were found on parental stress between the basic DC and NIDCAP group. Although not significant, the total stress scores in the NIDCAP intervention group were higher compared to the basic DC control group. The percentage of parents with a non-optimal parental stress score (> cut-off point 90th percentile, reference group of Dutch mothers) was approximately 10% for both groups and comparable to the percentage of parents scoring non optimal in the Dutch reference group.

NOSIK 1 year (range 1-6) ~	NIDCAP Mean (sd)	Basic DC Mean (sd)	NIDCAP-DC Difference # (99% CI diff.) #	NIDCAP % ≥ 90 perc. % (n)	Basic DC % ≥ 90 perc. % (n)	NIDCAP-DC Chi² ^ p-value
Total score Parent Domain	1.76 (.77)	1.75 (.76)	.04 (-.38;.45)			
Total score Child Domain	2.04 (1.00)	1.95 (.83)	.14 (-.37;.65)			
Total Stress score	1.92 (.86)	1.86 (.76)	.10 (-.35;.54)	10 % (6)	9 % (6)	.96

Table 4. Comparison NIDCAP and basic DC on parental stress at 1 year (NOSIK, short version).

\# Covariance analysis; difference (99% CI), corrected for the completion day after the age of 1 year, infant gender, gestational age, birth weight, CRIB and the age, educational level and country of birth of parents. N covariance: NIDCAP=58, basic DC=61

^ Chi-square test % scoring non optimal (p-value)

~ For all NOSIK scales: higher mean score represents more parental stress

Subgroup longer duration of intervention

Social relatedness was significantly better in the NIDCAP intervention group (Difference DC-C=0.27, 99%CI=0.02;.51, p=0.006) within a subgroup of 44 infants admitted > 45 days to the NICU in which the study took place (NIDCAP=21, DC=23).

Parental remarks on the care given to their child

Almost all parents expressed that they felt that the caregiving their child had received during admission had a positive effect. Thirty-one parents in the basic DC group (49% of the 63 parents that completed the questionnaire) and 42 parents in the NIDCAP group (65% of the 65 parents that completed the questionnaire) commented on the positive effect of the care their child received.

Some parents in the control group indicated that it was difficult for them to judge if this control care (basic DC) had any effects on their child but were overall positive with regards to the care their child had received and its effect on their infant. One parent specifically reported that the infant seemed to suffer less from unusual stimuli and that it seemed easy to apply and use the basic elements of developmental care in the unit.

Parents in the NIDCAP intervention group often attributed their child's positive behavior and development to the NIDCAP care. One parent for example stated that "He became a lot calmer and almost never cried. The reaction to NIDCAP was very noticeable". Parents furthermore indicated that the NIDCAP helped them during the admission of the infant and taught them how to observe their baby's behavioral cues. Parents commented: "It makes it easier for parents to gain and maintain contact with their infant" or "I got to know my baby really early" or "She is calm and feels safe, we now know when she is bothered by too many stimuli so we can remove them". Another parent stated that it made the period at the NICU easier for them. Parents indicated that they mainly observed the positive effects of NIDCAP during the period of admission. They, for example, reported: "During caregiving he seemed to appreciate the special care given to him but I find it difficult to comment on this" and "I mainly noticed the effect during admission, during the one-on-one contact with the nurse, but I do not think the effects last until now (1 year of age)".

Discussion

Parents expressed positive experiences with NIDCAP and reported positive effects on the comfort and well-being of their infant during admission. However, no significant effects were found of the NIDCAP intervention, compared to basic developmental care, on infant temperament at 9 months and infant behavior and parental stress at 1 year of the infant's corrected age. There was a tendency of improved social relatedness behavior as measured by the ITSEA at 1 year in the NIDCAP intervention group and this difference was significant in infants who received the intervention for more than 1.5 months.

The social relatedness domain of the ITSEA consists of three constructs, being social approach (i.e. "Is affectionate with loved ones"), relatedness (i.e. "Looks for you when upset") and social attention (i.e. "Looks right at you when you say his/her name"). A previous RCT [26] in the same Dutch NICU compared basic DC (standardized incubator covers and nests) with standard care (no forms of nests or covers). This RCT found a positive effect of basic DC on mastery motivation competence behavior at 1 year of age and no difference on social relatedness with 139 questionnaires (from the parents of 192 infants included at birth). One of the characteristics of the NIDCAP is that it focuses on the infants' behavioral cues for interaction with their caregivers and parents, which might have intensified the infants' social relatedness with their parents or changed the way parents perceived their child.

No effects were found of NIDCAP, compared to basic DC, on infant temperament at 9 months of age. A study by Keretes showed that the IBQ temperament scores of preterm infants at 6 and 12 months of age resembled the scores of term infants [27]. Furthermore, mean IBQ scores found in the current study resembled the scores of a sample of 9-12 months old infants (N=120) from a normal population in the USA [21]

The NIDCAP intervention did not improve parenting stress in the total study group and in the subgroup with a longer admission duration, as measured by a short version of the Dutch version (NOSIK) of the Parenting Stress Index (PSI) questionnaire. Although it was presumed that parenting stress of parents of a premature born infant is higher than of parents with a term infant, parental stress scores of the parents in both study groups resembled the scores of a reference group of mothers from the normal Dutch population.

The significant decrease of parental stress in the NIDCAP group in the three-center study by Als [13], as measured with the PSI questionnaire, was not found in the current Dutch study. One of the reasons could be that the average duration of the intervention in our study was relatively short, compared to the three-center study by Als [13], because infants admitted to the academic location of the NICU were transferred to a medium care unit of a local hospital when they became more stable. The three-center study by Als reported an average admission duration of 100 days until discharge while the current study showed a median admission duration of 36 (basic DC group) and 38 (NIDCAP group) days. Analysis of the infants admitted for more than 45 days showed a significant improvement of social relatedness at 1 year ($p=.006$) in the NIDCAP group. Stress scores were also a bit lower, although not significantly (data not shown) in the subgroup, instead of higher as in the total study group, which resembles the hypothesis of decreased stress. This suggests that a longer intervention duration might have a more positive effect on infant social relatedness behavior and parental stress.

Parents' remarks on the effect of the NIDCAP intervention at the end of the questionnaire indicated overall positive effects of NIDCAP on parents' experiences and the comfort and well-being of their infant during admission. However, no significant differences were found between the NIDCAP group and the basic DC group on the outcomes of the questionnaires. This suggests that future research should focus on the infant's comfort and pain-related infant behavior during admission or shortly after the intervention has ended, such as pain assessments [28] or measurements of infant behavior (for example: the Assessment of Preterm Infants' Behavior [29]).

This Dutch study furthermore showed that the effect of the NIDCAP intervention might be influenced by the Dutch setting and circumstances (i.e. the transfer policy), which suggests that it is difficult to generalize results from NIDCAP intervention studies. During the implementation of developmental care or NIDCAP in the Netherlands, it is important to ensure a continuation of developmental care by involving regional hospitals more and by evaluating the transition to another hospital and the transition after the infants are discharged to go home.

The NIDCAP training costs approximately 4.000 US$ per person and the training guide states that during training one needs to perform 20 observations and to observe 1 infant at the NICU biweekly or weekly from admission to discharge and one observation at the infant's home after discharge, which can be time-consuming [30].

Further research is needed to evaluate if positive outcomes can outweigh the cost and labor intensive characteristics of the NIDCAP intervention and a more complete costs-benefits analysis is warranted. Other medical and (neuro)developmental outcomes of the current study are needed for a complete representation of the effects of this study. Furthermore, this study shows that future study of an intervention with a longer duration and with other outcomes might be valuable. Until now, this study has showed a small positive effect on a domain of infant behavior at 1 year and found no other group differences. The positive effects reported by parents are also valuable and further evaluation of parents' experiences with NIDCAP and the experiences of the personnel at the NICU with NIDCAP might shed some light on outcomes that need to be explored in future randomized controlled trials.

This study suggests that it is valuable to implement a least several basic elements of developmental care in the Dutch setting, until other outcomes of future research are known. These basic aspects of developmental care might encompass the use of standardized nests and incubator covers, lower levels of sound, light and activity in the unit and clinical lessons for NICU personnel on infant behavior, based on the NIDCAP observational tool and the synactive theory of infant development.

Acknowledgements

We are grateful to the parents for taking the time and effort to fill in the questionnaires. We would also like to thank the medical and nursing staff at the Leiden University Medical Center and the Juliana Children's Hospital for their involvement in carrying out this study and ZONMW (grant 2100.0072) and the Health Care Efficiency Research Fund LUMC for funding this study.

References

1. Lau,R. & Morse,C.A. Stress experiences of parents with premature infants in a special care nursery. *Stress and Health* **19**, 69-78 (2003).

2. Singer,L.T. *et al.* Maternal psychological distress and parenting stress after the birth of a very low-birth-weight infant. *JAMA* **281**, 799-805 (1999).

3. Rautava,P., Lehtonen,L., Helenius,H. & Sillanpaa,M. Effect of newborn hospitalization on family and child behavior: a 12-year follow-up study. *Pediatrics* **111**, 277-283 (2003).

4. Holditch-Davis,D., Bartlett,T.R., Blickman,A.L. & Miles,M.S. Posttraumatic stress symptoms in mothers of premature infants. *J. Obstet. Gynecol. Neonatal Nurs.* **32**, 161-171 (2003).

5. Bhutta,A.T., Cleves,M.A., Casey,P.H., Cradock,M.M. & Anand,K.J. Cognitive and behavioral outcomes of school-aged children who were born preterm: a meta-analysis. *JAMA* **288**, 728-737 (2002).

6. Miceli,P.J. *et al.* Brief report: birth status, medical complications, and social environment: individual differences in development of preterm, very low birth weight infants. *J. Pediatr. Psychol.* **25**, 353-358 (2000).

7. Pierrehumbert,B., Nicole,A., Muller-Nix,C., Forcada-Guex,M. & Ansermet,F. Parental post-traumatic reactions after premature birth: implications for sleeping and eating problems in the infant. *Arch. Dis. Child Fetal Neonatal Ed* **88**, F400-F404 (2003).

8. Als,H. Developmental Interventions in the Neonatal Intensive Care Nursery. Goldson,E. (ed.), pp. 18-85 (Oxford University Press, New York,1999).

9. Als,H. Towards a synactive theory of development: Promise for the assessment of infant individuality. *Infant Mental Health Journal* **3**, 229-243 (1982).

10. Kleberg,A., Westrup,B. & Stjernqvist,K. Developmental outcome, child behaviour and mother-child interaction at 3 years of age following Newborn Individualized Developmental Care and Intervention Program (NIDCAP) intervention. *Early Hum. Dev.* **60**, 123-135 (2000).

11. Als,H. & Gilkerson,L. The role of relationship-based developmentally supportive newborn intensive care in strengthening outcome of preterm infants. *Semin. Perinatol.* **21**, 178-189 (1997).

12. Als,H. *et al.* Early experience alters brain function and structure. *Pediatrics* **113**, 846-857 (2004).

13. Als,H. *et al.* A three-center, randomized, controlled trial of individualized developmental care for very low birth weight preterm infants: medical, neurodevelopmental, parenting, and caregiving effects. *J. Dev. Behav. Pediatr.* **24**, 399-408 (2003).

14. Als,H. *et al.* Individualized developmental care for the very low-birth-weight preterm infant. Medical and neurofunctional effects. *JAMA* **272**, 853-858 (1994).

15. Mouradian,L.E. & Als,H. The influence of neonatal intensive care unit caregiving practices on motor functioning of preterm infants. *Am. J. Occup. Ther.* **48**, 527-533 (1994).

16. Buehler,D.M., Als,H., Duffy,F.H., McAnulty,G.B. & Liederman,J. Effectiveness of individualized developmental care for low-risk preterm infants: behavioral and electrophysiologic evidence. *Pediatrics* **96**, 923-932 (1995).

17. Fleisher,B.E. *et al.* Individualized developmental care for very-low-birth-weight premature infants. *Clin. Pediatr. (Phila)* **34**, 523-529 (1995).

18. Westrup,B., Kleberg,A., von Eichwald,K., Stjernqvist,K. & Lagercrantz,H. A randomized, controlled trial to evaluate the effects of the newborn individualized developmental care and assessment program in a Swedish setting. *Pediatrics* **105**, 66-72 (2000).

19. Westrup,B., Bohm,B., Lagercrantz,H. & Stjernqvist,K. Preschool outcome in children born very prematurely and cared for according to the Newborn Individualized Developmental Care and Assessment Program (NIDCAP). *Acta Paediatr.* **93**, 498-507 (2004).

20. Symington,A. & Pinelli,J. Developmental care for promoting development and preventing morbidity in preterm infants. *Cochrane. Database. Syst. Rev.* CD001814 (2006).

21. Gartstein,M.A. & Rothbart,M.K. Studying infant temperament via the Revised Infant Behavior Questionnaire. *Infant Behavior & Development* **26**, 64-86 (2003).

22. Carter,A.S., Briggs-Gowan,M.J., Jones,S.M. & Little,T.D. The Infant-Toddler Social and Emotional Assessment (ITSEA): factor structure, reliability, and validity. *J. Abnorm. Child Psychol.* **31**, 495-514 (2003).

23. de Brock,A.J.L.L., Vermulst,A.A., Gerris,J.R.M. & Abidin,R.R. NOSI - Nijmeegse Ouderlijke Stress Index, Handleiding experimentele versie [NOSI- Nijmegen Parenting Stress Index, Manual experimental version]. Swets en Zeitlinger, Lisse (1992).

24. The International Neonatal Network. The CRIB (clinical risk index for babies) score: a tool for assessing initial neonatal risk and comparing performance of neonatal intensive care units. *Lancet* **342**, 193-198 (1993).

25. Abidin,R.R. Parenting Stress Index. Pediatric Psychology Press, Charlottesville (1983).

26. van der Pal,S.M. *et al.* Very Preterm Infant's Behavior at 1 and 2 Years of Age and Parental Stress Following Basic Developmental Care. *Manuscript submitted for publication* (2007).

27. Kerestes,G. Maternal ratings of temperamental characteristics of healthy premature infants are indistinguishable from those of full-term infants. *Croat. Med. J.* **46**, 36-44 (2005).

28. Mathew,P.J. & Mathew,J.L. Assessment and management of pain in infants. *Postgrad. Med. J.* **79**, 438-443 (2003).

29. Als,H., Butler,S., Kosta,S. & McAnulty,G. The Assessment of Preterm Infants' Behavior (APIB): furthering the understanding and measurement of neurodevelopmental competence in preterm and full-term infants. *Ment. Retard. Dev. Disabil. Res. Rev.* **11**, 94-102 (2005).

30. Als,H. Program Guide - newborn individualized developmental care and assessment program (NIDCAP): an education and training program for health care proffesionals. The Children's Medical Centre Corporation, Boston (1996).

CHAPTER 6

Staff opinions regarding the Newborn Individualized Developmental Care and Assessment Program (NIDCAP)

YLVIA M. VAN DER PAL
ELESTE M. MAGUIRE
ASKIA LE CESSIE
YLVIA VEEN
AN MAARTEN WIT
RANS J. WALTHER
EANET BRUIL

CCEPTED FOR PUBLICATION IN EARLY HUMAN DEVELOPMENT

Abstract

Objective

To explore (para)medical and nursing staff opinions regarding the Newborn Individualized Developmental Care and Assessment Program (NIDCAP) implementation in two Dutch Neonatal Intensive Care Units (NICU's).

Methods

A questionnaire was send to the personnel of 2 Dutch NICU's after implementing NIDCAP. The questionnaire measured: a) the perceived impact of NIDCAP on several NICU conditions, b) attitudes, subjective norm and perceived behavioral control, knowledge and abilities of using the NIDCAP method (based on the Theory of Planned Behavior) and c) training interest, requirements, information sources and the relevance of the NIDCAP method for different groups of NICU patients.

Data

Seventy-four percent (124 out of 168) of the questionnaires were returned and respondents were in general positive with regards to NIDCAP and felt that using NIDCAP is fulfilling and leads to improvement in the infant's development, health and well-being. The NIDCAP was however also thought to be time-consuming and might worsen job conditions. Although respondents indicated sufficient abilities and knowledge they also indicated a need for ongoing information and guidance. The use of the NIDCAP method during caregiving was related to a higher perceived behavioral control, intention and subjective norm (R square=0.49). The nursing staff, compared to the medical staff, had a more positive attitude (p=.004), higher perceived behavioral control (p=.004) and perceived a more positive impact of NIDCAP on NICU conditions (p=.008).

Conclusion

When implementing NIDCAP the monitoring of intentions and attitudes, ongoing practical NIDCAP guidance and information, time-efficiency and the involvement of different disciplines are of importance.

Introduction

The Newborn Individualized Developmental Care and Assessment Program (NIDCAP®) is being introduced and used increasingly in Neonatal Intensive Care Units (NICU's) as a more individualized and family-based way of caregiving. Studies have shown that NIDCAP results in positive outcomes such as improved short term medical outcomes [1-4] , better behavioral performance as measured with the Assessment of Preterm Behaviour (APIB) [1,2,5-7], improved cognitive developmental outcome [2,3,5,8], a positive impact on behavior [9], reduced hospital charges [3], less parental stress [1] and improved brain function and altered brain structure [5]. Reviews that report on these NIDCAP studies call for more trials with large samples sizes to study the long-term effects of NIDCAP in multiple settings [10-12].

NIDCAP uses an observational tool based on the Synactive Theory of Development where the preterm infant's behavior is observed along four channels of communication, being: autonomic, motor, state organization and attention-interaction. The infant's efforts at self-regulation and interaction are observed through approach and avoidance behaviors and the infant's efforts and individual goals and recommendations for caregiving are discussed with parents and other caregivers [8,13-15]. An example of an individual recommendation is to give time-outs when the infant shows individual signs of stress or fatigue. The NICU environment and care are also critically reviewed to meet the infant's developmental needs. Examples of basic recommendations are: reduced light, sound and activity levels in the NICU, for example by using incubator covers, and support of positioning, for example by using standardized nests.

Implementing NIDCAP in a NICU is very intensive and asks for changes in the NICU environment, care, expertise and attitudes. Staff may, in return for their effort, experience positive results in the infants and their parents. Als and Gilkerson [14] stated that because NIDCAP is process-guided and relationship-based and not procedure-based, it can be difficult to implement NIDCAP in a NICU which focuses on medical protocols and caregiving routines. Furthermore, NIDCAP is system-orientated and implemented in an existing organisational structure, social system, and nursing and medical culture which can influence the success of the implementation [14]. When promoting the use of NIDCAP at a NICU, variables predicting the behavior and intention to use NIDCAP are of importance. In the Theory of Planned Behavior (TOPB) [16,17] Ajzen states that intention predicts behavior and intention is thought to be influenced by the individual's attitude towards the behavior, the subjective norm held by important people in their surroundings and how they perceive their control, knowledge and abilities with regards to the behavior.

A study evaluating the NIDCAP implementation in a Swedish setting examined staff opinions and concluded that NIDCAP was in general well received by nursing staff, neonatologists and parents [18,19]. Staff indicated improvements in their ability to assess the infant, the infant's well-being and the opportunities for and quality of parental attachment. This study mainly focused on the impact of NIDCAP on several NICU conditions.

The current study aims to explore nursing and (para)medical staff's opinions concerning the use of NIDCAP in a Dutch NICU at two locations, which could lead to recommendations for future NIDCAP implementation strategies. This study furthermore aims to explore the determinants influencing the intention to use the NIDCAP method in the NICU.

Methods

NIDCAP implementation and subjects

The implementation process of the NIDCAP in a Dutch Neonatal Intensive Care Unit (NICU) at two locations (the Leiden University Medical Center (LUMC) in Leiden and the Juliana Children's Hospital in the Hague) was carried out through a 4 year two-phased randomized controlled trial and was done in steps for research purposes. During the first two years (phase 1), basic developmental care was implemented by using standardized incubator covers to decrease light, sound and activity levels and nesting for positional support. During the last two years (phase 2), official NIDCAP observations and guidance were implemented under the supervision of a NIDCAP certified psychologist and 5 certified nurses. In addition, clinical NIDCAP lessons were given for nurses who were assigned to take care of the infants receiving NIDCAP care in the randomized controlled trial. After 4 years of implementation a questionnaire concerning the implementation of NIDCAP was sent to the home addresses of the (para)medical and nursing staff of the two locations. Before the questionnaires were constructed, interviews with several staff members were done for orientation. The questionnaires were not numbered to guarantee anonymity of the respondents. As a result it was not possible to track which staff members did not return the questionnaire. General reminder notes were distributed in both locations to remind personnel to return the questionnaire.

Questionnaire

The questionnaire constructed for this study measured a) the perceived impact of NIDCAP on several NICU conditions, as used by Westrup in the Swedish NIDCAP study [18,19], b) attitudes, subjective norm and perceived behavioral control, based on the Theory of Planned Behavior [16,17], c) training interest, requirements, information sources and the relevance of the NIDCAP method for different groups of NICU patients questions, and d) background information such as gender, age and work experience of the respondents.

The Swedish questionnaire [18,19] measuring the impact of NIDCAP included 25 NICU related conditions. Staff was asked to indicate their perception of the impact NIDCAP on these conditions on a 5 point Likert scale (1=condition became worse, 2=slightly worse, 3=the same, 4= slightly better, 5=better). In the current study the total scale has a Cronbach's alpha reliability score of 0.92. The items are displayed in Figure 1.

Nineteen items were based on the TOPB [16,17] and were divided over the five factors of the TOPB (Figure 2) being: behavior (1 item), intention (2 items) attitude (8 items), perceived behavioral control (4 items) and subjective norm (4 items). Mean factor scores were calculated for all items belonging to a factor. The items were formulated as statements using a 5 point Likert scale with answer categories ranging from 1 (I totally disagree) to 5 (I totally agree). In this study, alpha scores for the factors were reasonably good (α's ranged from 0.70 to 0.83, and alpha was 0.53 for subjective norm). Half of the attitude items (nr. 2, 4, 5 and 6) were formulated in a negative way and half in a positive way. When the total attitude factor was calculated, the 4 negatively formulated items were recoded so a higher attitude factor score represented a positive attitude.

Other relevant questions that were thought to be important during the implementation of NIDCAP, for example the respondent's interest to be NIDCAP trained and the requirements for NIDCAP implementation, were added to the questionnaire. All items could be answered by both active users and non-users of the NIDCAP method.

Data analysis

Mean scores and 95% confidence intervals of the means were calculated for the items based on the Theory of Planned Behavior and the items measuring the impact of NIDCAP on NICU conditions. For analysis of the perceived impact of NIDCAP on NICU conditions only the respondents that indicated working for 4 years or more at the two NICU's (when NIDCAP was implemented) were included, because they were thought to be most able to detect change at the NICU. The valid percentages per answer category were calculated for the all other items, for example when describing training interest.

A backward linear regression analysis with all respondents was carried out to check in which way the intention to use the NIDCAP method during caregiving (dependent factor, mean score of two questions on a 5 point Likert scale) was influenced by the respondents' characteristics (block 1; gender, age, being a nurse or neonatologist (or resident), the hospital the respondent works at and the years of work experience), and the factors of the TOBP and the total perceived impact of all NICU conditions combined (block 2; attitude, subjective norm, perceived behavioral control and the total perceived impact). A second similar linear regression analysis was carried out with the actual behavior (the use of the NIDCAP method during caregiving) as dependent factor and with intention as an additional independent variable. The assumptions for multiple regression were checked.

A comparison between the scores of the nursing staff and medical staff on attitude, perceived behavioral control, subjective norm and mean perceived impact of NIDCAP on the NICU conditions, was done using a two sample t-test.

Results

Respondents

Initially, 168 questionnaires were sent to the home addresses of the NICU personnel of a Dutch NICU at two locations and 124 questionnaires were completed resulting in a return rate of 74% (Table 1). The characteristics of the respondents are displayed in Table 1.

Return rate	Nurses	76% (93 out of 122)
	Neonatologists/pediatricians (in training)	58% (18 out of 31)
	Physical therapists	60% (3 out of 5)
	Lab technicians of NICU	100% (5 out of 5)
	Psychologists	100% (1 out of 1)
	Social workers	50% (2 out of 4)
	Unknown	2
Gender	Male	12% (n=15)
	Female	88% (n=107)
Age	20-35 years	41% (n=50)
	35-50 years	50% (n=61)
	> 50 years	9% (n=11)
NICU	Leiden University Medical Center	51% (n=62)
	Juliana Children's Hospital	47% (n=57)
	At both NICU's	2% (n=3)
Experience	In a NICU (mean)	8.23 years
	In the current NICU (mean)	7.74 years
	> 4 years at current NICU	62% (77)

Table 1. Return rate per profession and characteristics of respondents

Familiarity with NIDCAP, information sources and requirements
Table 2 shows the familiarity of the respondents with NIDCAP, the main NIDCAP information sources and requirements for implementing NIDCAP. More than half of the respondents (63%) were very familiar with NIDCAP. Only 3% of the respondents indicated being only fairly familiar with NIDCAP, which indicates that all respondents were at least somewhat familiar with the NIDCAP construct and related behavior discussed in the questionnaire. The randomized controlled trial at both hospitals and the presentations and education of the NIDCAP team were most often reported as sources of NIDCAP information (Table 2).

" I am familiar with NIDCAP " N=121				
Totally disagree	Fairly disagree	Partly agree/disagree	Fairly agree	Totally agree
0%	3%	7%	28%	63%

Informed through:	N = 123	Requirements implementation:	N = 120
Randomized Controlled Trial	93%	More education	50%
Presentations/education NIDCAP team	60%	More time during caregiving	48%
Clinical lessons	39%	More NIDCAP trained personnel	41%
Education related to profession	37%	More personnel in general	39%
Conversation with colleagues	29%	More materials (nests and covers)	33%
Work meetings/consultations	26%		
Profession related education	25%		
Conferences/symposia	24%		
Daily patients' visits	11%		

Table 2. NIDCAP familiarity, information sources and requirements for implementation.

Fifty percent of the respondents indicated that more education about NIDCAP is a necessary requirement when implementing NIDCAP (Table 2) and 48% indicated that more time during caregiving is needed. Other requirements indicated were: more multi-disciplinary involvement (especially more involvement of management personnel and physicians), enough standardized NIDCAP supporting materials (nests and covers) and parent facilities and more guidance by a NIDCAP trained staff member during caregiving. One respondent suggested assigning a special nurse to provide NIDCAP support to infants during caregiving. When asked for additional remarks at the final page of the questionnaire, some respondents indicated a need for up to date and continuing clinical lessons with more detailed explanation on the individual application of materials, handling during caregiving and the individual behavioral signals of infants. They also indicated a need for assistance and instruction from the NIDCAP trained staff on the work floor and suggested providing NIDCAP handbooks for parents and nurses or physicians.

Perceived impact of NIDCAP on NICU conditions

The mean scores and their 95% confidence intervals regarding the perceived impact of NIDCAP on NICU conditions (worse-better) are summarized in Figure 1 for the 77 respondents working for more than 4 years at one of the two locations. Overall, most respondents reported improvement on the NICU related conditions, as a result of NIDCAP. Most improvement (highest scores) was found on the items "..the infant's well-being during hospital stay" (mean=4.92) and "..the infant's well-being due to the reduction of light" (mean=4.79). Neutral or even negative scores were found on the items "..my job satisfaction due to the demand for reduced light" (mean=3.14) and "The individual NIDCAP care plans have influenced the conditions for fulfilling my tasks" (mean=2.85).

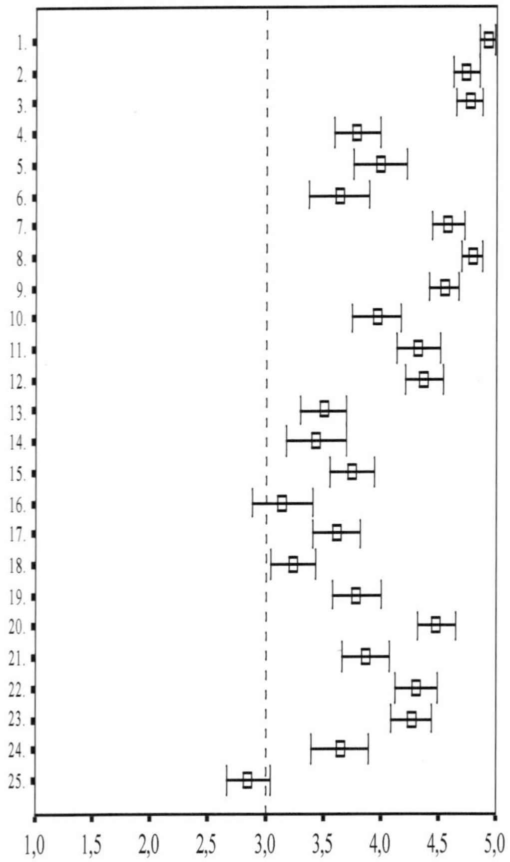

As a result of NIDCAP ... has become worse/unchanged/better when compared to conventional care:

1... the infant's well-being during its hospital stay (mean=4.92)
2... my capability to influence the infant's well-being (mean=4.74)
3... the infant's opportunities to rest and sleep (mean=4.76)
4... the infant's ability to cope with enteral feeding (mean=3.79)
5... the safety of the infant (mean=3.99)
6... my capability to assess the infant's condition (mean=3.64)
7... the infant's well-being due to the demands on reduction in sound (mean=4.58)
8... the infant's well-being due to the demands on reduction of light (mean=4.79)
9... the infant's well-being due to the demands on reduction in activity (mean=4.55)
10... the presence of the parents at the infant's bedside (mean=3.96)
11... the parents' way of caring for their infant (mean=4.32)
12... the parents' attachment to their infant (mean=4.37)
13... my own confidence in my professional role (mean=3.50)
14... the conditions for performing my job (mean=3.43)
15... my job satisfaction due to the demand for a reduced sound level (mean=3.75)
16... my job satisfaction due to the demand for reduced light (mean=3.14)
17... my job satisfaction due to the demand for reduced activity (mean=3.62)
18... my working conditions in general (mean=3.24)
19... my satisfaction with my work in general (mean=3.79)

The individual NIDCAP care plans have influenced ...

20... the infant's opportunities to rest and sleep (mean=4.48)
21... the presence of the parents at the infant's bedside (mean=3.87)
22... the parents' way of care-giving (mean=4.31)
23... the parents' attachment to their infant (mean=4.27)
24... my opportunities to adequately assess the infant's condition (mean=3.65)
25... the conditions for fulfilling my tasks (mean=2.85)

1 = worse, 2 = slightly worse, 3 = no change, 4 = slightly better, 5 = better

Figure 1. Change in NICU conditions as a result of NIDCAP (95% C.I. of Mean), respondents working ≥ 4 years at NICU (N=71-77).

Attitude, perceived behavioral control and subjective norm (TOPB)
The mean scores for the attitude, perceived behavioral control, subjective norm and intention for all respondents are displayed in Figure 2. The attitude questions show that, in general, respondents had a positive attitude towards using the NIDCAP method and on average considered the use of the NIDCAP method as enjoyable (mean=4.31), fulfilling (mean=4.19). They viewed the use of NIDCAP as an improvement of care (mean=4.52) and an improvement of the infants' health and development (recoded mean=4.20). However, they also felt that it was time-consuming (mean=3.46). Respondents indicated having enough knowledge (mean=3.76) and abilities (mean=3.71) to use the NIDCAP method during caregiving. However, they indicated that it was not their own choice to use the NIDCAP method during caregiving (mean=2.28). The subjective norm of the nursing and medical staff in general about using the NIDCAP method during caregiving was high indicating that respondents felt a strong subjective norm from others (nurses or medical specialists) that they should use the NIDCAP (general subjective norm perceived from nurses mean=4.13 / from medical specialists mean=3.34). Respondents did indicate that the opinion of others was not important for them in their choice to use the NIDCAP method (mean=2.45). Overall, the respondents intended to use the NIDCAP method during caregiving (mean = 3.95 and 4.24) and most of the respondents agreed (mean = 4.03) with the statement of already using the NIDCAP method during caregiving (Figure 2). Of the 4 respondents that did not use NIDCAP 75% (n=3) did have the intention to use NIDCAP in the future and of the 84 respondents that indicated using NIDCAP during caregiving 5% (n=4) did not indicated the intention to continue to use NIDCAP.

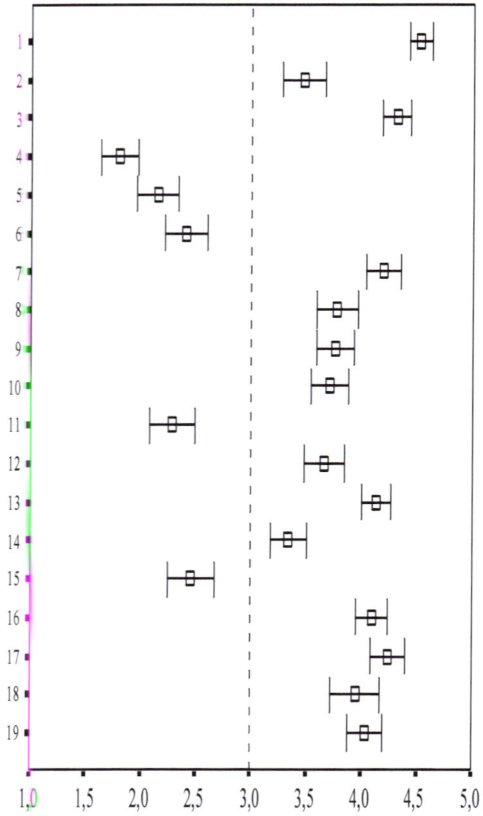

Attitude:

1. Using NIDCAP during caregiving is an improvement of our care (mean=4.52)
2. Using NIDCAP during caregiving is time consuming (mean=3.46)
3. It is enjoyable to use NIDCAP during caregiving (mean=4.31)
4. Using NIDCAP during caregiving does not lead to an improvement in the health and development of the infants (mean=1.80)
5. The NICU care is good enough without NIDCAP (mean=2.14)
6. Using NIDCAP during caregiving is not practical when carrying out my job (mean=2.40)
7. It is self-fulfilling to use NIDCAP during caregiving (mean=4.19)
8. Using NIDCAP during caregiving is good for my job progress (mean=3.77)

Perceived Behavioral Control:

9. I have enough NIDCAP knowledge to use NIDCAP during caregiving (mean=3.76)
10. I have enough abilities to use NIDCAP during caregiving (mean=3.71)
11. It is my own choice if I want to use NIDCAP during caregiving (mean=2.28)
12. It is not difficult for me to use NIDCAP during caregiving if I want to (mean=3.66)

Subjective Norm

13. The nurses think the NIDCAP method should be used during caregiving (mean=4.13)
14. The medical specialists think the NIDCAP method should be used during caregiving (mean=3.34)
15. The opinion of others is important to me in my choice to use NIDCAP during caregiving (mean=2.45)
16. I expect others to use NIDCAP during caregiving (mean=4.09)

Intention

17. I would like to use the NIDCAP method during caregiving (mean=4.24)
18. I am planning to use the NIDCAP method during caregiving (mean=3.95)

Behavior

19. I use the NIDCAP method during caregiving (mean=4.03)

1 = totally disagree, 2 = fairly disagree, 3 = fairly agree/disagree, 4 = fairly agree, 5 = totally agree

Figure 2. Agreement with Theory of Planned Behavior statements (95% Confidence Interval of Mean) all respondents (N=116-123).

Factors influencing the use of the NIDCAP method

Four variables remained in a final model (R square =0.40) predicting a higher intention to use the NIDCAP method during caregiving, namely (in order of their contribution): a higher subjective norm, a higher attitude, a higher perceived behavioral control and lower age. In the final model, predicting a higher actual use of the NIDCAP method during caregiving (R square = 0.49), three variables remained, namely: a higher perceived behavioral control, a higher intention and a higher subjective norm. The two final models and the standardized beta per variable are summarized in Figure 3.

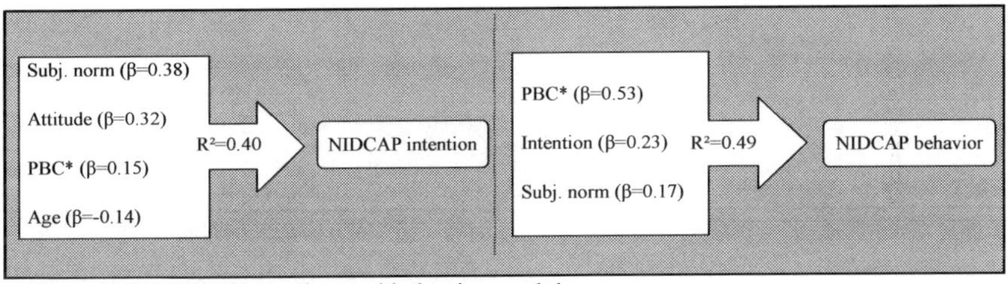

Figure 3. NIDCAP intention and behavior models

* PCB = perceived behavioral control

P-values standardized beta's:

Model 1: Subj.norm + Attitude p=<0.001, PBC p=0.08, Age p=0.08

Model 2: PCB p=<0.001, Intention p=0.007, Subj.norm p=0.04

Table 3 shows that medical staff members, compared to nursing staff, had a significantly less positive attitude towards NIDCAP (p=.004), perceived less behavioral control regarding the use of NIDCAP (p=.004) and indicated less improvement in the NICU as a result of NIDCAP (p=.008).

Factors (range 0-5)	Nursing staff (n=92) mean(sd)	Medical staff (n=18) mean(sd)	Difference (95% CI)
Attitude	3.91 (.60)	3.44 (.62)	.46 (.15;.78)*
Perceived behavioral control	3.42 (.69)	2.90 (.70)	.52 (.17;.87)*
Subjective norm	3.46 (.56)	3.71 (.67)	-.25 (-.54;.05)
NICU conditions (worse-better)	4.01 (.48)	3.69 (.34)	.32 (.08;.56)*
Intention	4.16 (.92)	3.72 (.89)	.43 (-.04;.90)
Behavior (use NIDCAP method)	4.03 (.88)	3.78 (.65)	.26 (-.18;.69)

Table 3. Difference between the medical and nursing staff and the NIDCAP team and other nurses at LUMC NICU.

* p<.01

Necessity of NIDCAP observations, training interest and general remarks

Respondents recommended the NIDCAP observations and guidance most for preterm infants with a gestational age below 30 and 32 weeks (Figure 4) and only recommend the NIDCAP observations in some cases for very ill term infants, infants born small for gestational age and infants with a gestational age below 37 weeks. Respondents indicated that the observations might, in addition, be helpful for irritable or drug-addicted infants and infants with certain problems, for example difficulties with breastfeeding. Respondents furthermore suggested doing only one observation during a specific caregiving interaction when an individual infant showed a specific problem.

One psychologist and 7 nurses were officially NIDCAP trained when they completed the questionnaire. Fifty-eight percent of the other respondents were not interested in doing the official NIDCAP training themselves, 24% was not sure and 17% did want to do the NIDCAP training. The main reasons for not aspiring to do the NIDCAP training were: other priorities, too time-consuming and too much work to write the long NIDCAP reports. The main reasons for interest in the NIDCAP training were to know more about infant behavior and to improve behavior observation abilities during caregiving.

There was a possibility for respondents to provide additional remarks about the NIDCAP implementation in their NICU on the last page. Several respondents indicated that the complete NIDCAP reports were very extensive and too much work to write. Furthermore, the recommendations following the observations were often thought to overlap. Because of this, respondents felt that the observation reports were not read most of the times. They felt that more in depth and up-to-date information about the infant's behavior in the medical record would make the extensive NIDCAP reports superfluous. Furthermore, respondents wanted to be informed about the long-term effects of NIDCAP on the infants' health and development.

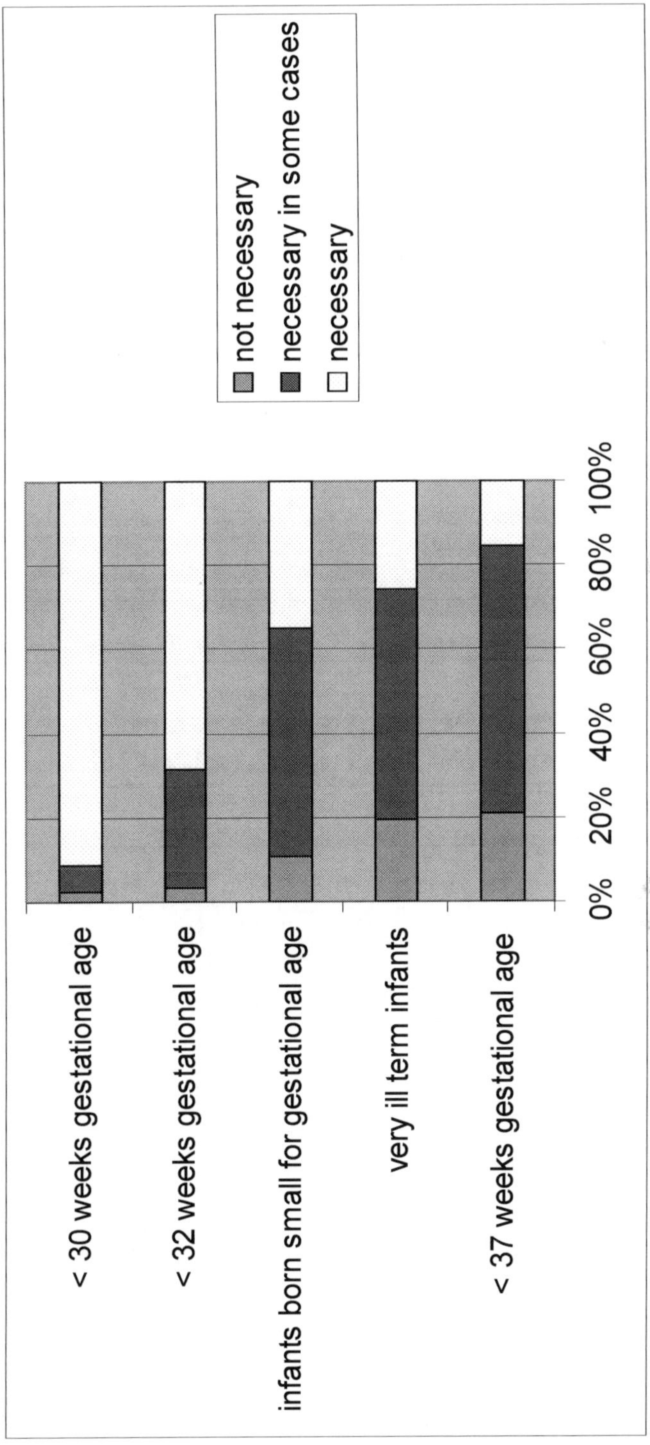

Figure 4. Necessity of NIDCAP observations and guidance (N=113-118)

Discussion

Opinions regarding NIDCAP implementation

This study shows overall positive attitudes of the nursing and (para)medical staff regarding the NIDCAP implementation in a NICU at two locations in the Netherlands. While the perceived benefits of NIDCAP were high, especially concerning the infants' well being, the perceived impact regarding the staff's job conditions was neutral or at some points even negative. For example, the demand to reduce light was considered an improvement for the infant's well-being but could also cause less job satisfaction. The mean scores on the impact of NIDCAP on several NICU conditions and the difference found between the impact of NIDCAP on the infant's well-being and the respondents' work conditions are comparable to the results found in the Swedish study [18,19]. A study by Heermann and Wilson, using structured interviews with open questions, also found both positive and negative results of implementing developmental care [20]. Nurses in this study reported positive experiences as a result of the increasing involvement of parents and parents' ability to participate in care. These nurses, however, also reported feelings of intimidation and loss of control. Als has previously recommended that 10% of the nursing staff needs to be NIDCAP certified to successfully implement the NIDCAP in a NICU [14]. In the current study 17% of the respondents indicated wanting to do the official NIDCAP training, from which can be concluded that NIDCAP training interest at this NICU matches the recommendation of 10% of nursing staff being trained.

Theoretic framework.

Respondents indicated that they used the NIDCAP method during caregiving most of the time. This behavior was influenced most by higher perceived behavioral control, subjective norm and intention. The perceived behavioral control influenced the actual behavior of using the NIDCAP more than the intention to use NIDCAP. Perceived behavioral control therefore seemed important for transitioning from the intention to use the NIDCAP method to the actual behavior. A review study by Godin and Kok [21] showed that the TOPB was well applicable for different health related behaviors (for example exercising, clinical screening or addictions). The current study shows that the

TOPB is also applicable for caregiving related behavior. Being a member of the nursing staff (compared to the medical staff) had a positive effect on attitude, perceived behavioral control and perceived improvement on NICU conditions. A difference between nurses and medical specialists was that nurses received more clinical NIDCAP lessons. Job related priorities and interests might have also influenced these differences.

Methodological considerations.

Presumably selection bias did not influence the results because the return rate was good. The medical staff was somewhat underrepresented in comparison to the other disciplines. Unfortunately, we had no baseline measurements of the opinions of NICU staff on NIDCAP before the implementation, which might have shed more light on the prediction of intention and behavior over time. When exploring opinions of the impact of NIDCAP on the NICU conditions, we only included the respondents working for 4 years or more at the hospital to make sure they were able to report on the change over time due to the implementation of NIDCAP.

Recommendations regarding NIDCAP implementation.

Continuous and up to date information.

When implementing NIDCAP it is important to respond to the need for ongoing information. It is also important to supply staff with the results of recent studies regarding the effects of developmental care and NIDCAP.

Continuous clinical lessons and practical guidance.

In the current study respondents indicated to have enough NIDCAP knowledge and abilities. However, they still felt a need for more and ongoing practical NIDCAP education and practical guidance during caregiving. Continuous clinical lessons and practical assistance during caregiving are needed. A suggestion is to introduce a developmental care or NIDCAP notebook or an email box where staff can indicate on which subjects they need additional practical information or if they want individual instructions during caregiving.

Multi-disciplinary approach.

The subjective norm about NIDCAP in the NICU needs to be considered when implementing NIDCAP. There seems to be a discrepancy between medical and nursing staff on several points. Respondents indicated that especially the nursing staff felt they should use the NIDCAP method during caregiving and indicated that medical staff and management personnel should show more involvement. When forming a NIDCAP team, all relevant disciplines should be included, such as physicians, managing personnel, psychologists, social workers and a parent representative (to include parent opinions). Involving physicians is important because they handle infants frequently and communicate the condition of the infant to the parents. Adapted clinical lessons for medical specialists highlighting NIDCAP information relevant for medical specialists are recommended.

Possibilities to improve job conditions.

Because the implementation of NIDCAP might worsen job conditions, for example through the reduction of light, possibilities should be reviewed to make sure the infant's well-being improves but not at the expense of the job conditions of the staff. One option is to create a separate area for other nursing activities, such as charting, apart from the area where the infants sleep and where the demands for reduced light, sound and activity may benefit the infants.

Review possibilities for efficiency.

One of the reasons why respondents were not interested in the official NIDCAP training was that they felt the NIDCAP reports were too extensive and overlapped most of the time. It is advisable to summarize the most important recommendations for an individual infant and place them next to the incubator, primarily as a short reminder for the medical and nursing staff. This worked well in the NICU described in this study. However, the reports of the observations also contain new and interesting information for parents who are not familiar with the neonatal caregiving. Furthermore, the reports contain important additional information for staff about the infant's individual goals and behavior. The first report might therefore need to address all relevant topics belonging to the official NIDCAP observations [14], while the following reports might be shortened updates with the most relevant findings and not too many repetitions. Possibilities for extra time during caregiving and time efficiency should also be reviewed.

The recommendations for the implementation of NIDCAP as stated here resemble those described by Als and Gilkerson [14], i.e.: the assignment of a developmental staff position (one full-time developmental specialist, one full-time developmental nurse and a parent representative), ongoing NIDCAP training, leadership involvement, a multi-disciplinary developmental team and opportunities for a reflective process with regularly scheduled supervision.

In conclusion, staff opinions and experience regarding NIDCAP are positive in a Dutch NICU at two locations included in this study. The decision to implement NIDCAP should be evaluated by the individual units and based on the outcomes from future research. When deciding to implement NIDCAP the (para)medical and nursing staff's opinions and suggestions should be well monitored and it is important to supply information and ongoing practical guidance. Time-efficiency and the involvement of different disciplines are also of importance.

Acknowledgements

We are indebted to the nursing and (para)medical staff of the Leiden University Medical Center and the Juliana Children's Hospital for taking the time and effort to fill in the questionnaires. We would also like to thank ZONMW (grant 2100.0072) and the Health Care Efficiency Research Fund LUMC for funding this study.

References

1. Als,H. *et al.* A three-center, randomized, controlled trial of individualized developmental care for very low birth weight preterm infants: medical, neurodevelopmental, parenting, and caregiving effects. *J. Dev. Behav. Pediatr.* **24**, 399-408 (2003).

2. Als,H. *et al.* Individualized developmental care for the very low-birth-weight preterm infant. Medical and neurofunctional effects. *JAMA* **272**, 853-858 (1994).

3. Fleisher,B.E. *et al.* Individualized developmental care for very-low-birth-weight premature infants. *Clin. Pediatr. (Phila)* **34**, 523-529 (1995).

4. Westrup,B., Kleberg,A., von Eichwald,K., Stjernqvist,K. & Lagercrantz,H. A randomized, controlled trial to evaluate the effects of the newborn individualized developmental care and assessment program in a Swedish setting. *Pediatrics* **105**, 66-72 (2000).

5. Als,H. *et al.* Early experience alters brain function and structure. *Pediatrics* **113**, 846-857 (2004).

6. Buehler,D.M., Als,H., Duffy,F.H., McAnulty,G.B. & Liederman,J. Effectiveness of individualized developmental care for low-risk preterm infants: behavioral and electrophysiologic evidence. *Pediatrics* **96**, 923-932 (1995).

7. Mouradian,L.E. & Als,H. The influence of neonatal intensive care unit caregiving practices on motor functioning of preterm infants. *Am. J. Occup. Ther.* **48**, 527-533 (1994).

8. Kleberg,A., Westrup,B. & Stjernqvist,K. Developmental outcome, child behaviour and mother-child interaction at 3 years of age following Newborn Individualized Developmental Care and Intervention Program (NIDCAP) intervention. *Early Hum. Dev.* **60**, 123-135 (2000).

9. Westrup,B., Bohm,B., Lagercrantz,H. & Stjernqvist,K. Preschool outcome in children born very prematurely and cared for according to the Newborn Individualized Developmental Care and Assessment Program (NIDCAP). *Acta Paediatr.* **93**, 498-507 (2004).

10. McCarton,C.M., Wallace,I.F. & Bennett,F.C. Preventive interventions with low birth weight premature infants: an evaluation of their success. *Semin. Perinatol.* **19**, 330-340 (1995).

11. Sizun,J. & Westrup,B. Early developmental care for preterm neonates: a call for more research. *Arch. Dis. Child Fetal Neonatal Ed* **89**, F384-F388 (2004).

12. Symington,A. & Pinelli,J. Developmental care for promoting development and preventing morbidity in preterm infants. *Cochrane. Database. Syst. Rev.* CD001814 (2006).

13. Als,H. Towards a synactive theory of development: Promise for the assessment of infant individuality. *Infant Mental Health Journal* **3**, 229-243 (1982).

14. Als,H. & Gilkerson,L. The role of relationship-based developmentally supportive newborn intensive care in strengthening outcome of preterm infants. *Semin. Perinatol.* **21**, 178-189 (1997).

15. Als,H. Developmental Interventions in the Neonatal Intensive Care Nursery. Goldson,E. (ed.), pp. 18-85 (Oxford University Press, New York,1999).

16. Ajzen,I. The Theory of Planned Behavior. *Organizational Behavior and Human Decision Processes* **50**, 179-211 (1991).

17. Ajzen,I. & Madden,T.J. Prediction of Goal-Directed Behavior: Attitudes, Intentions and Perceived Behavioral Control. *Journal of Experimental Social Psychology* **22**, 453-474 (1986).

18. Westrup,B., Stjernqvist,K., Kleberg,A., Hellstrom-Westas,L. & Lagercrantz,H. Neonatal individualized care in practice: a Swedish experience. *Semin. Neonatol.* **7**, 447-457 (2002).

19. Westrup,B. *et al.* Evaluation of the Newborn Individualized Developmental Care and Assessment Program (NIDCAP) in a Swedish setting. *Prenatal and Neonatal Medicine* **2**, 366-375 (1997).

20. Heermann,J.A. & Wilson,M.E. Nurses' experiences working with families in an NICU during implementation of family-focused developmental care. *Neonatal Netw.* **19**, 23-29 (2000).

21. Godin,G. & Kok,G. The theory of planned behavior: a review of its applications to health-related behaviors. *Am. J. Health Promot.* **11**, 87-98 (1996).

CHAPTER 7

General discussion

Discussion

Developmental care interventions that focus on the individuality of the infant, family and environment, such as the Newborn Individualized Developmental Care and Assessment Program (NIDCAP) are recently being integrated in Dutch Neonatal Intensive Care Units (NICU) in various forms. This thesis reported on the effects of a basic form of Developmental Care and the effects of the NIDCAP intervention, with individual observations and guidance, on the behavior and health related quality of life (HRQoL) of very preterm infants born < 32 weeks of gestation and their parent's experiences and stress. This thesis furthermore explored the nursing and (para)medical staff's experiences with the implementation of NIDCAP in their unit.

The study consisted of two consecutive Randomized Controlled Trials (RCT). The first trial measured the effect of basic developmental care (basic DC: using standardized nests to support positioning and incubator covers to protect the infant from sound, light and activity coming from the nursery), compared to standard care. The second trial explored the effect of the NIDCAP intervention (individualized observations and guidance by a developmental specialist), compared to basic DC. We expected the basic form of developmental care to positively influence health and behavior because of the stimulation of rest through the protection from environmental stimuli and the support of positioning. We also thought that basic DC would decrease parental stress because parents might perceive their infant as being more comfortable in the nests and underneath the incubator covers. We expected the individual characteristics of the NIDCAP observations and guidance in the second trial to further intensify these positive effects, especially on parental stress. The somatic and developmental outcomes of the infant (the medical outcomes during admission and the neurological and developmental examinations at 1 and 2 years of age) will be reported and discussed in another thesis.

Effect of developmental care on parent's experiences and stress

The first trial revealed that basic DC did not decrease parental stress during admission or at 1 or 2 years of the infant's age and did not increase parental confidence or perceived nurse support during admission. The more individualized and family-based characteristics of the NIDCAP observations and the guidance by a NIDCAP trained developmental specialist during the second RCT had no effects on parental stress, confidence and perceived nurse support during the infant's admission and parental stress at 1 and 2 years of the infant's age.

As in other studies that measure parental stress of parents of preterm born infants, we found higher stress levels of mothers compared to fathers during the infant's admission. In the second trial, we found a decrease in the difference between the stress levels of mothers and fathers in the NIDCAP group, compared to the basic DC group. The effects of higher paternal stress levels on infants and the family have, to our knowledge, not been studied before. A study by Miles et al. concluded that the higher stress levels of mothers, especially on the parent role alteration stressors (as also found in the current study), suggests that mothers are more affected by the loss of the caretaking role than fathers [1]. Jackson and colleagues [2] interviewed parents and concluded that it was often difficult for fathers to get leave from work and that they had no choice but to leave the care to the nursing and medical staff. The aim of the NIDCAP to equally involve both parents in the caregiving and to approach them as the main caregivers could have led to higher stress levels in fathers, which became more similar to maternal stress levels.

Effect of developmental care on health-related quality of life

No significant effects were found of basic DC in the first RCT and the NIDCAP observations and guidance in the second RCT on the infant's health-related quality of life at 1 year. To our knowledge HRQoL has not been previously used as an outcome to measure the effect of a developmental care intervention. Our hypothesis was that the nests and incubator covers would increase the infant's opportunities for rest and, as a result, would improve the infant's health and health-related quality of life. Most children had optimal HRQoL scores (score of 100), which did not leave much of a window of opportunity to increase HRQoL.

Effect of developmental care on infant behavior

In the first RCT, a positive effect was found of basic DC on the competence behavior scale and its subscale mastery motivation of the ITSEA infant behavior questionnaire [3], completed at 1 year of corrected age. This indicates that the infants that received basic Developmental Care (standardized incubator covers and nests) showed more curiosity, persistence and enjoyment with small accomplishments and that they were more often well-behaved and obedient at 1 year of corrected age, compared to the infants that received standard care. The effect on infant competence behavior might be caused by the protective characteristics of the nests and covers that allowed the infants to rest and gain more control over their behavior. No effects were found on problem behavior at 1 and 2 year. At 2 years of age the CBCL [4] was given to measure problem behavior. This questionnaire does not measure competence behavior and therefore it was not possible to measure if the positive effect on competence behavior found at 1 year had persisted at 2 years of age.

In the second RCT, social relatedness behavior was better in the NIDCAP intervention group (compared to the basic DC control group) at 1 year of the infant's age, especially when the intervention duration was longer than 1.5 months. The social relatedness scale encompasses social approach ("Is affectionate with loved ones"), relatedness ("Looks for you when upset") and social attention ("Looks at you when you say his/her name"). One of the characteristics of the NIDCAP is that it focuses on the infants' behavioral cues for interaction with their caregivers and parents, which might have intensified the infants' social relatedness with their parents. No effects were found on infant temperament at 9 months and infant problem behavior at 1 year of age during the second RCT. The difference found in the first RCT on infant competence behavior at 1 year of age, was not found in the second RCT. In both trials we found no effects on problem behavior and we only found an effect of both interventions on one behavior domain of the ITSEA, which encompasses only a part the behavioral spectrum of the infants.

Comparison to other NIDCAP studies

Previous studies show positive outcomes of the NIDCAP intervention [5-13]. A recent study using a three-center randomized controlled trial [6] found promising effects of the NIDCAP intervention on different outcomes, such as shorter duration of parental feeding, transition to full oral feeding, intensive care and hospitalization; lower incidence of necrotizing enterocolitis; reduced discharge ages and hospital charges; improved weight, length and head circumferences. This study found several effects on behavior at two weeks after the expected due date, such as enhanced autonomic, motor, state, attention and self-regulatory functioning on the Assessment of Preterm Infants' Behavior (APIB) [14] and reduced need for facilitation during the APIB. The three-center study also found lowered family stress on the Parenting Stress Index and enhanced appreciation of the infant. A recent study by Als and colleagues [7] with infants 28-33 weeks gestation and free of known developmental risks found enhanced brain function and structure (on neurobehavior assessment, developmental test, EEG and MRI) in the NIDCAP intervention group (n=16). This study in the USA found no effects on medical outcome variables at 2 weeks and 9 months of corrected age [7].

In contrast to what we expected, our study found no significant, clinically relevant differences between the basic developmental care and NIDCAP group and controls on parental stress and the infants' problem behavior and health-related quality of life. We were therefore not able to replicate the positive findings on parental stress and behavior found in the three center NIDCAP study [6]. In comparison to the current study, the mean gestational age at birth in the sample of the three center NIDCAP study was lower and the hospital stay and stay at the NICU where the intervention took place was noticeably longer.

Two NIDCAP studies took place in Sweden [15] and it is possible that the situation of a European country is more comparable to the Dutch situation. The first study consisted of two consecutive study periods of control (n=21) and intervention (n=21) care. This study found no significant differences in requirement for ventilatory support or weight gain for preterm infants with a birth weight below 1500 grams [15]. At 3 years of corrected age, improved hearing-speech development, improved child behavior and improved child communication regarding mother-child interaction was found in the NIDCAP group [10]. A second study, with a randomized controlled design, was performed a year later with 25 infants born below 32 weeks of gestation and in need of ventilatory support. This Swedish RCT found less days of continuous positive airway pressure (CPAP) and oxygen was withdrawn at a younger post conceptual age in the NIDCAP intervention group [12]. This second Swedish study also found improved mental development at 1 year of corrected age [16] and a positive impact on infant behavior at 5,5 years of corrected age [13]. However, the sample size of the Swedish RCT was small because inclusion was terminated before the required number of infants was included because of spill over effects and other methodological reasons. The Swedish study recently reported on mothers' perception of NIDCAP [17] and concluded that although mothers in the NIDCAP group perceived more nurse support and closeness to their infant, they also expressed more anxiety. The authors suggested that higher anxiety might be a sign of early bonding [17].This finding is comparable to our finding of increased parental stress after basic DC and increased paternal stress after NIDCAP.

Meta-analysis of the NIDCAP data shows only small benefits of the NIDCAP intervention on oxygen requirements during admission [18,19]. A recent Cochrane review [18] discussed that a large number of outcomes showed no or conflicting effects and that the main effects were mostly found using small RCT's and could not be replicated in other small trials. Another review [19] emphasized that the methodological quality of NIDCAP studies is poor and a cost-benefits analysis seems appropriate because of the expensive and labor intensive characteristics of the NIDCAP intervention. Sizun and Westrup [20] have called for more research and argue that a large randomized controlled trial with multiple centers, long term neurobehavioral and developmental outcomes and a cost-effectiveness analysis seems of importance.

In the context of these reviews, the current study provides important additional information regarding the outcomes of two large consecutive RCT's measuring the effect of a basic form of developmental care and the additional effect of the individualized aspects and guidance of the NIDCAP intervention in the Netherlands until 2 year of the infant's corrected age. This RCT found only small differences on competence behavior and social relatedness behavior and was not able to replicate the findings of reduced parental stress levels on the Parenting Stress Index questionnaire found in the three-center study in the USA. Also, no effects were found on the health-related quality of life of the infants. The NIDCAP reviews and meta-analysis call for studies in different settings and the current study shows that the NIDCAP has limited benefits in the Dutch setting with regards to the outcomes described in this thesis. Other infant outcomes of the current study need to be reviewed before a complete representation of effects can be given.

Evaluation of parents and staff experiences

Next to the results based on standardized questionnaires, the experiences of parents and the nursing and medical staff with NIDCAP are also of importance when evaluating the effect of NIDCAP. In this context, parents were asked to complete an open-ended question on the final page of the questionnaire at 1 year where they were able to indicate if the care their child had received had positive or negative effects. Parents overall indicated positive effects on the well-being of their infant during admission and on their own experiences during the admission of their infant.

An evaluation of the experiences of the nursing and (para)medical staff after the implementation of NIDCAP showed that the staff reported positive attitudes and experiences towards NIDCAP. Staff members felt that using NIDCAP is fulfilling and leads to improvements in the infant's development, health and well-being. The main problem with the NIDCAP observations seemed to be its time-consuming characteristics. In addition, some standard developmental care recommendations might worsen job conditions (for example because of reduced light levels at the unit). The nursing staff was more positive compared to the medical staff. The use of the NIDCAP method during caregiving was related to a higher intention, perceived behavioral control (their perceived control over using NIDCAP during caregiving) and subjective norm (the norm about using NIDCAP in the unit and the perceived importance of these norms). Although respondents indicated sufficient abilities and knowledge they also indicated a need for ongoing information and guidance.

The evaluation of staff opinions led to the following recommendations regarding the implementation of NIDCAP: easy access to continuous and up to date information about NIDCAP and NIDCAP related issues and research, continuous clinical lessons and practical guidance, a multi-disciplinary approach and a multi-disciplinary NIDCAP team, possibilities to improve and discuss NIDCAP related job conditions (such as the reduction in light) and possibilities to review improving (time)efficiency. The applicability of these recommendations is dependent on the characteristics and available resources in the unit.

In conclusion, parents and the nursing and medical staff reported positive experiences with NIDCAP, especially with regards to the infant's comfort and wellbeing during caregiving, but this does not result in significant differences on the questionnaires given during admission and at 1 and 2 years of the infant's corrected age.

Research implications: Duration of intervention

The infants in this study were admitted for on average approximately 1 month to the NICU where the study took place. The NICU's in Dutch academic hospitals, such as the unit in Leiden, are mainly specialized in intensive care and infants are transferred to a regional hospital as soon as they become more stable. Therefore the duration of admission was sometimes short. We found that the positive effect of the NIDCAP intervention on social relatedness at 1 year was more profound if the duration of intervention was longer. This raises the question if the duration of the intervention in this study was long enough to measure significant effects. The three-center NIDCAP trial in the USA [6] found positive effects on parental stress and infant behavior with infants who were admitted for a more extended period of time (mean admission duration until discharge of approximately 100 days). These positive outcomes were not found in the current study. Interventions during admission with home visits after discharge have also found promising effects on parental stress [21] and infant problem solving and behavior ratings [22].

Following the results of the current study, compared with the results of other studies, it is recommendable to study a NIDCAP based intervention with a longer duration. In the context of the Dutch transfer policy of the NICU's in the academic hospitals, it is important to make sure that the special care is being continued in the regional hospitals. Regional developmental care or NIDCAP teams might enhance the communication between the academic and regional hospitals. In addition, a study exploring the effects of a developmental care based intervention including home visits after discharge seems recommendable. It is not difficult to imagine that parents might appreciate some guidance and recommendations after discharge, when they are left on their own to take care of their infant in the different circumstances at home. The need for home visits from the parent's point of view could be evaluated with a short qualitative parent questionnaire or interview.

Research implications: Outcome measures

This thesis explored parent outcomes during admission and parental stress and infant behavior and health-related quality of life at 1 and 2 years of the infant's corrected age with standardized questionnaires. Both parents and the nursing and (para)medical staff observed a positive effect of NIDCAP on the well-being and comfort of the infant during admission. This effect observed by staff and parents is not confirmed by the results on the outcomes measured with the standardized questionnaires. The well-being and behavior of the infants during admission was not measured in the current study. The observed effect on the infant's well-being by parents and staff suggest that it might be worthwhile to measure infant comfort through infant pain assessment [23] or by using the NIDCAP behavior observation sheets [24]. Infant behavior might also be actively tested during admission by administering, for example, the Assessment of Preterm Infants' Behavior (APIB) [14], which is used as an outcome measure in the three center NIDCAP study.

This study shows that additional qualitative interviews among parents and the nursing and (para)medical staff might provide important additional information about relevant outcomes for future research, such as infant comfort during admission. The outcomes of a randomized controlled trial with standardized questionnaires, should not be interpreted as the sole outcome on which decisions of implementation are based. Outcomes during or shortly after an intervention, also seem of importance because the infant and parents might then experience the effect of the intervention most profoundly. The other outcomes of the current study (somatic and developmental outcomes of the infant at 1 and 2 years of age) will be discussed in another thesis and are of importance for a complete representation of effects.

Qualitative questionnaires and interviews can also be of importance to evaluate the specific experiences and needs of parents and nursing and (para)medical staff. The outcomes could provide information about which aspects of early intervention and NIDCAP are the least or the most important to implement if one would only want to implement some aspects of the NIDCAP.

Research implications: Cost analysis

The study described in this thesis only found small benefits of the NIDCAP on infant behavior. The Cochrane review of previous Developmental Care studies concluded that research needs to focus more on providing cost-benefits information [18]. The three center NIDCAP trial [6] and the study on the effect of NIDCAP by Fleisher [9] did find lower hospital charges in the NIDCAP group. However, a review on NIDCAP by Jacobs [19] discussed that the charges for developmental assessments, the salary for a developmental specialist and the costs for training should be taken into account when studying the effect of NIDCAP. The training costs are approximately 4.000 US$ per person. Furthermore, the NIDCAP program guide states that 2 salaried positions (2 FTE) should be assured for a developmental specialist and a developmental care nurse educator [25]. The labor-intensive characteristics of the NIDCAP training and observations and guidance can also be costly. During training, one needs to perform 20 observations and to observe 1 infant at the NICU biweekly or weekly from admission until discharge and one observation at the infants home [25]. Observations should be done weekly or biweekly and an observation (including writing the report) usually costs approximately a working day. Besides further research on other possible benefits of NIDCAP, further research regarding these costs seems appropriate.

Methodological considerations: Study design

Although randomization seemed to have resulted in comparable groups regarding the parent and child characteristics, covariate analysis was done with the parent and child characteristics as covariates. This was done for a more precise estimation of the differences between the groups on the outcome variables. Some questionnaires were missing in the covariance analysis because parents did not fill in their age or educational level. For comparison, in the context of selection bias, we performed t-tests which resulted in approximately the same significant differences of the total sample and the sample in the covariance analysis. The non-significant differences were also non-significant in the two sample t-tests with the total sample. When calculating the mean scores of the scales the scale score was a missing value if more than 30% of the items were not completed. This was done to make sure that most aspects (items) of the construct were completed and the scale score still resembled the whole construct measured. Furthermore, we corrected for multiple comparisons, which increases the possibility of finding a significant difference, by using a $p<.01$ as the level of significance.

When designing a randomized controlled trial to explore the effect of the NIDCAP intervention, it seems impossible to make the intervention double blind. It is always clearly visible for parents and the nursing and medical staff to which study group infant belongs. The outcomes described in this thesis mainly depend on parent reports through standardized questionnaires and therefore could be influenced by some bias because parents know which treatment their child received. The visible aspects of the intervention were, however, also thought to be the main reasons for a positive effect on one of the outcomes, namely parental stress.

The inclusion of infants for the NIDCAP study in Sweden was stopped before the required amount of infants was reached because of a spill-over effect [12]. The inclusion of infants in the Swedish RCT study took longer than expected and spill-over effect occurred because nurses were convinced of the benefits of NIDCAP and indicated feeling uncomfortable taking care of the control infants. Because we included infants born < 32 weeks admitted to a large NICU with two locations in the current study, we were able to include a large number of infants in two consecutive trials over only 4 years of time. Furthermore, because we did not implement NIDCAP at once but in two consecutive steps during the two RCT's and it was not an "all or nothing" intervention, we expect to have minimised to effect of spill-over. The absence of the nests and covers in the control groups in the first trial and the absence of the NIDCAP observations and guidance in the second trial were adopted and respected by nursing and medical staff for research purposes. Nursing staff did indicate feeling relieved when the inclusion for the trials was finished and all infants were allowed the same treatment.

In the Netherlands a cut-off point was formulated for the treatment of preterm infants which indicates that only infants born > 25 weeks of gestation receive active treatment. This results in a population of infants with a higher gestational age at the NICU's in the Netherlands compared to, for example, the USA. The NIDCAP observations and guidance might work best within infants born with a low gestational age. The two NIDCAP studies in Sweden, which used different inclusion criteria, showed a difference in effect from which the researchers concluded that the impact of the NIDCAP intervention on medical outcomes might be correlated to the degree of prematurity and the severity of illness [15].

Because the study design consisted of two consecutive RCT's it was difficult to compare the standard care control group in the first trial with the NIDCAP intervention group in the second trial, which might have led to additional information. The basic developmental care groups in both trials were also not completely comparable regarding the infant's health condition at birth (infants in the second phase had a better mean CRIB clinical risk score and higher birth weight). Furthermore, the basic developmental care groups in both trials were not comparable on certain outcomes while both groups had received basic developmental care.

Additional analysis showed that of the couples that completed the questionnaire at admission but did not complete the questionnaire at 1 year (of both RCT's taken together), the mothers had reported significantly (p=.013) more stress during admission compared to the mothers that completed both questionnaires. The stress of fathers during admission did not differ among the couples that did or did not complete the questionnaire at 1 year. This indicates that we lost the group of most stressful mothers. Further analysis within this group that was lost at 1 year, showed that the control and intervention groups in both RCT's had comparable maternal stress levels during admission (data not shown). We therefore concluded that the loss of the more stressed mothers had no large effect on the final results of our RCT's.

This study found a small effect of the NIDCAP intervention on competence behavior, which is only a part of the behavioral spectrum. In the context of multiple comparisons, one should be cautious when interpreting the significant differences. It might be difficult for interventions at the NICU to obtain statistical significant effects on outcomes that do not differ from the general population. Some outcomes correspond with problems that are primarily related to the circumstances of the preterm birth. For example, the health-related quality of life of preterm infants at 1 year was lower, compared to infant born at term [26] on the stomach, lungs and eating problems scales, which seem related to the preterm birth. Health-related quality of life was furthermore already optimal for most infants in both groups which does not leave much of a window of opportunity to improve quality of life. McCarton and colleagues [27] reviewed preventive interventions for low birth weight infants and suggested that many infants develop within normal limits and might never have the need for corrective intervention programs. In this context, competence behavior might be more easily improved. This seems to be a relevant outcome on which a positive effect was found in the current study.

The support by social worker is standard and equally available for parents from all social economic levels in the Netherlands. This Dutch study also showed that the effect of the NIDCAP intervention seems influenced by the

Dutch setting and circumstances (i.e. the transfer policy). This suggests that it is difficult to generalize results from NIDCAP intervention studies and meta-analysis as a guideline for implementation in other settings.

The study design described in this thesis also has its strengths. Two large randomized samples were obtained to measure the effect of both a basic form of developmental care and the more extensive NIDCAP intervention. Furthermore, most infants remained in the study during follow up at 1 and 2 years of age.

Practical implications

The evaluation of staff opinions in a Dutch NICU led to several recommendations for the implementation of NIDCAP or developmental care in a NICU, being: easy access to continuous and up to date information, continuous clinical lessons, practical guidance, a multi-disciplinary approach and a multi-disciplinary NIDCAP team. In addition, it is necessary to minimize the possible negative effects of NIDCAP on job conditions and possibilities to improve (time)efficiency should be reviewed. The applicability of these recommendations depends on the specific characteristics and available resources of the unit and it is therefore recommendable to evaluate the consequences and possibilities per individual unit. Secondly, the decrease in the difference in stress levels of fathers and mothers, with mothers experiencing more stress than fathers, suggests that during the implementation it is important to evaluate and stimulate the involvement of fathers.

The current study found improved competence behavior of infants that had received the basic elements of developmental care (standardized nests and incubator covers). The standardized nests and covers are easy to implement and the theory of the reduction of external stimuli by creating an environment comparable to the womb seems logical. However, when implementing aspects of developmental care, it is important to involve regional hospitals more to ensure the continuation of the special care and information for parents.

The extensive NIDCAP intervention improved the infant's social relatedness behavior. This finding seems to relate to the aspect of the NIDCAP that it focuses on the infants' behavioral cues for interaction with their caregivers and parents, which might have intensified the infants' social relatedness with their parents. Parents and nurses furthermore indicated a visible improvement on the well-being of the infants that received NIDCAP during admission. However, the NIDCAP intervention also costs money and time and is labor intensive.

Further research is needed to evaluate if positive outcomes can outweigh the cost and labor intensive characteristics of the NIDCAP intervention and a more complete costs-benefits analysis is warranted. Other medical and (neuro)developmental outcomes of the current study are needed for a complete representation of the effects of this study. Furthermore, this study shows that future study of an intervention with a longer duration and with other outcomes might be valuable. Until now, this study has showed a small positive effect on a domain of infant behavior at 1 year and found no other group differences. The positive effects and experiences with NIDCAP reported by parents and personnel at the NICU, are also valuable and further evaluation of parents' experiences with NIDCAP and the experiences of the personnel at the NICU with NIDCAP might shed some light on outcomes that need to be explored in future randomized controlled trials.

This thesis suggests that it is valuable to implement a least several basic elements of developmental care in the Dutch setting, until other outcomes of future research are known. These basic aspects of Developmental Care can encompass the use of standardized nests and incubator covers and lower levels of sound, light and activity in the unit. In addition, some basic recommendations and clinical lessons on infant behavior, based on the NIDCAP observational tool and the synactive theory of infant development, need to be formulated. Evaluation of the importance and applicability of different aspects of the NIDCAP might lead to the development of a less intensive NIDCAP based intervention.

References

1. Miles,M.S., Funk,S.G. & Kasper,M.A. The stress response of mothers and fathers of preterm infants. *Res. Nurs. Health* **15**, 261-269 (1992).

2. Jackson,K., Ternestedt,B.M. & Schollin,J. From alienation to familiarity: experiences of mothers and fathers of preterm infants. *J. Adv. Nurs.* **43**, 120-129 (2003).

3. Carter,A.S., Briggs-Gowan,M.J., Jones,S.M. & Little,T.D. The Infant-Toddler Social and Emotional Assessment (ITSEA): factor structure, reliability, and validity. *J. Abnorm. Child Psychol.* **31**, 495-514 (2003).

4. Achenbach,T.M., Edelbrock,C. & Howell,C.T. Empirically based assessment of the behavioral/emotional problems of 2- and 3- year-old children. *J. Abnorm. Child Psychol.* **15**, 629-650 (1987).

5. Als,H. *et al.* Individualized developmental care for the very low-birth-weight preterm infant. Medical and neurofunctional effects. *JAMA* **272**, 853-858 (1994).

6. Als,H. *et al.* A three-center, randomized, controlled trial of individualized developmental care for very low birth weight preterm infants: medical, neurodevelopmental, parenting, and caregiving effects. *J. Dev. Behav. Pediatr.* **24**, 399-408 (2003).

7. Als,H. *et al.* Early experience alters brain function and structure. *Pediatrics* **113**, 846-857 (2004).

8. Buehler,D.M., Als,H., Duffy,F.H., McAnulty,G.B. & Liederman,J. Effectiveness of individualized developmental care for low-risk preterm infants: behavioral and electrophysiologic evidence. *Pediatrics* **96**, 923-932 (1995).

9. Fleisher,B.E. *et al.* Individualized developmental care for very-low-birth-weight premature infants. *Clin. Pediatr. (Phila)* **34**, 523-529 (1995).

10. Kleberg,A., Westrup,B. & Stjernqvist,K. Developmental outcome, child behaviour and mother-child interaction at 3 years of age following Newborn Individualized Developmental Care and Intervention Program (NIDCAP) intervention. *Early Hum. Dev.* **60**, 123-135 (2000).

11. Mouradian,L.E. & Als,H. The influence of neonatal intensive care unit caregiving practices on motor functioning of preterm infants. *Am. J. Occup. Ther.* **48**, 527-533 (1994).

12. Westrup,B., Kleberg,A., von Eichwald,K., Stjernqvist,K. & Lagercrantz,H. A randomized, controlled trial to evaluate the effects of the newborn individualized developmental care and assessment program in a Swedish setting. *Pediatrics* **105**, 66-72 (2000).

13. Westrup,B., Bohm,B., Lagercrantz,H. & Stjernqvist,K. Preschool outcome in children born very prematurely and cared for according to the Newborn Individualized Developmental Care and Assessment Program (NIDCAP). *Acta Paediatr.* **93**, 498-507 (2004).

14. Als,H., Butler,S., Kosta,S. & McAnulty,G. The Assessment of Preterm Infants' Behavior (APIB): furthering the understanding and measurement of neurodevelopmental competence in preterm and full-term infants. *Ment. Retard. Dev. Disabil. Res. Rev.* **11**, 94-102 (2005).

15. Westrup,B., Stjernqvist,K., Kleberg,A., Hellstrom-Westas,L. & Lagercrantz,H. Neonatal individualized care in practice: a Swedish experience. *Semin. Neonatol.* 7, 447-457 (2002).

16. Kleberg,A., Westrup,B., Stjernqvist,K. & Lagercrantz,H. Indications of improved cognitive development at one year of age among infants born very prematurely who received care based on the Newborn Individualized Developmental Care and Assessment Program (NIDCAP). *Early Hum. Dev.* **68**, 83-91 (2002).

17. Kleberg,A., Hellstrom-Westas,L. & Widstrom,A.M. Mothers' perception of Newborn Individualized Developmental Care and Assessment Program (NIDCAP) as compared to conventional care. *Early Hum. Dev.* (2006).

18. Symington,A. & Pinelli,J. Developmental care for promoting development and preventing morbidity in preterm infants. *Cochrane. Database. Syst. Rev.* CD001814 (2006).

19. Jacobs,S.E., Sokol,J. & Ohlsson,A. The Newborn Individualized Developmental Care and Assessment Program is not supported by meta-analyses of the data. *J. Pediatr.* **140**, 699-706 (2002).

20. Sizun,J. & Westrup,B. Early developmental care for preterm neonates: a call for more research. *Arch. Dis. Child Fetal Neonatal Ed* **89**, F384-F388 (2004).

21. Kaaresen,P.I., Ronning,J.A., Ulvund,S.E. & Dahl,L.B. A Randomized, Controlled Trial of the Effectiveness of an Early-Intervention Program in Reducing Parenting Stress After Preterm Birth. *Pediatrics* **118**, e9-e19 (2006).

22. Gardner,J.M., Walker,S.P., Powell,C.A. & Grantham-McGregor,S. A randomized controlled trial of a home-visiting intervention on cognition and behavior in term low birth weight infants. *J. Pediatr.* **143**, 634-639 (2003).

23. Mathew,P.J. & Mathew,J.L. Assessment and management of pain in infants. *Postgrad. Med. J.* **79**, 438-443 (2003).

24. Als,H. Developmental Interventions in the Neonatal Intensive Care Nursery. Goldson,E. (ed.), pp. 18-85 (Oxford University Press, New York,1999).

25. Als,H. Program Guide - newborn individualized developmental care and assessment program (NIDCAP): an education and training program for health care proffesionals. The Children's Medical Centre Corporation, Boston (1996).

26. Stoelhorst,G. Development, Quality of Life and Behavior at 2 Years of Age in Very Preterm Infants (PhD thesis). Leiden University Medical Centre, Leiden (2003).

27. McCarton,C.M., Wallace,I.F. & Bennett,F.C. Preventive interventions with low birth weight premature infants: an evaluation of their success. *Semin. Perinatol.* **19**, 330-340 (1995).

SUMMARY

Summary

Focus in neonatal care giving has shifted to a more individualized and family-centered approach. In the 1980's Heidelise Als introduced individualized developmental care, which is based on the Synactive Theory of Development. This theory looks at the infant's individual behavior in specific circumstances and looks at the infant's emotional state transition, developmental stage and efforts at self-regulation and interaction through observed approach and avoidance behavior. This theory has led to some basic developmental care based recommendations for neonatal care such as reduced activity, light and sound levels in the infant's environment (for example by using incubator covers) and the support of the infant's (flexed) positioning (for example by the use of standardized nests).

The Newborn Individualized Developmental Care and Assessment Program (NIDCAP) is an intervention which uses a standardized observation tool. Nursing and (para)medical staff need special training to use this tool. The observation and recommendations are discussed with parents and other caregivers and parents are stimulated to become more actively involved in the caregiving process. Studies in the USA and Sweden have shown promising results but reviews on developmental care call for more large randomized controlled trials in multiple settings. Because of the labor intensive and costly characteristics of the NIDCAP, hospitals often implement the basic non-individualized recommendations of developmental care (reduced activity, light and sound and positioning support) as a first step before training personnel.

This thesis described the outcomes of two consecutive randomized controlled trials (inclusion period from 2000-2004: first trial included 192 infants and the second trial included 168 infants) in a Dutch level III NICU at two locations (Leiden and The Hague). The first trial explored the effect of basic developmental care (the use of standardized incubator covers and standardized nests) compared to standard care. The second trial explored the effect of the more individualized NIDCAP intervention compared to basic developmental care. This thesis focused on the effects of these two interventions on the infant's behavior and health-related quality of live and the experiences of their parents and the nursing and (para)medical staff.

Chapter 2 of this thesis described the effect of basic developmental care, and the more individualized NIDCAP intervention on parental stress, confidence and perceived nursing support during the admission of the infant (completed questionnaires: RCT1=133 and RCT2=150). The NIDCAP intervention tended to increase paternal stress (decrease of the higher stress levels of mother versus father, p=.03), possibly as a result of increased involvement of fathers. No effects were found of both interventions on the overall stress level, confidence and perceived nurse support of mother and father.

The effect of basic developmental care and the NIDCAP intervention on the infant's Health-Related Quality of Life (HRQoL) at 1 year of the infant's age, corrected for prematurity, was described in **chapter 3**. HRQoL scores were good to optimal for most infants (completed questionnaires RCT1=136, RCT2=128). Neither basic developmental care nor the NIDCAP intervention improved HRQoL of very preterm infants at 1 year, as reported by parents.

In **chapter 4** we explored the effect of basic Developmental Care on the behavior of very preterm infants and parental stress at 1 and 2 years of corrected age (completed questionnaires at 1 year = 139 and at 2 years = 133), compared to standard care. We found a significant positive effect on the infant's competence behavior at 1 year (p=.009), especially on mastery motivation (p=.002) related competence behavior. No significant effects were found on parental stress and problem behavior. We therefore concluded that the basic elements of developmental care have a positive influence on the child's competence behavior at 1 year of age.

Chapter 5 described the effects of the more individualized NIDCAP intervention, compared to basic developmental care, on parental stress and infant behavior (completed questionnaires = 128) and temperament (completed questionnaires = 134) during the first year. The NIDCAP tended to improve social relatedness behavior at 1 year (p=.011), especially when the duration of admission in the NICU where the study took place was longer (duration of the intervention > 1.5 months, $p=.006$). Parents overall indicated positive effects on their own experiences and the well-being of their infant during admission but this did not significantly improve the infant's temperament or parental stress at 1 year.

An evaluation of the opinions of the (para)medical and nursing staff regarding the NIDCAP implementation during the two RCT's in the Neonatal Intensive Care Unit in Leiden and The Hague was described in **chapter 6**. We concluded that, in general, staff members (N=124) were positive with regards to NIDCAP. Staff reported observing improvement in the infants' well-being as a result of the NIDCAP caregiving. However, the NIDCAP was considered to be time-consuming and might worsen some job conditions. Respondents furthermore indicated a need for ongoing information and guidance. The nursing staff seemed to be more positive about NIDCAP, compared to the medical staff ($p=.004$). These findings led to the following recommendations with regards to the implementation of NIDCAP: easy access to continuous and up to date information about NIDCAP related issues and research, continuous clinical lessons and practical guidance, a multi-disciplinary approach and a multi-disciplinary NIDCAP team, possibilities to improve and discuss NIDCAP related job conditions and possibilities to review improving (time)efficiency.

Chapter 7 discussed the implications for future research and the implementation of developmental care in the light of the results described in this thesis. We only found small effects on infant behavior in a Dutch setting on the outcomes discussed in this thesis. However, both parents and staff report positive effect on the comfort and well-being of the infant during admission. A study on the effects of NIDCAP with a longer duration and possibly home visits in the Dutch setting would be an interesting sequel of the current study. Before decisions can be made with regards to the implementation of the NIDCAP, other outcomes (medical and (neuro)developmental) in other settings and a thorough cost-benefit analysis should demonstrate if future positive outcomes outweigh the costs. Until then, it seems advisable to implement the less intensive basic elements of developmental care and to formulate other basic recommendations for care giving and for the training of personnel, based on the NIDCAP observational tool and the synactive theory of infant development.

SAMENVATTING

Samenvatting

Een vroeggeboorte heeft een grote impact op het kind en zijn ouders, zelfs na de opname op de neonatologieafdeling. Te vroeg geboren kinderen laten meer gedragsproblemen zien dan op tijd geboren kinderen en hun ouders ervaren meer ouderlijke stress dan ouders van op tijd geboren kinderen. Daarom is de nadruk in de neonatale zorg meer komen te liggen op de individuele zorg van het kind en het gezin.

In de jaren tachtig introduceerde Heidelise Als de individuele ontwikkelingsgerichte zorg, die gebaseerd is op de synactieve theorie van de ontwikkeling. Deze theorie kijkt naar het kind in zijn individuele omgeving en kijkt naar zijn emotionele toestand en ontwikkelingsfase en zijn pogingen tot zelfregulatie en interactie met behulp van toenadering en ontwijkend gedrag. Deze theorie heeft geleid tot basisaanbevelingen voor de neonatologieafdeling, gebaseerd op ontwikkelingsgerichte zorg. Deze basisaanbevelingen bestaan uit het verminderen van het geluid, het licht en de activiteit op de afdeling (bijvoorbeeld met behulp van couveusehoezen) en het ondersteunen van een ronde gebogen houding van het kind (bijvoorbeeld met behulp van speciale nestjes).

Het Newborn Individualized Developmental Care and Assessment Program (het NIDCAP) is een interventie waarbij, naast de boven beschreven algemene aspecten van ontwikkelingsgerichte zorg, het gedrag van het kind geobserveerd wordt door speciaal getraind personeel. De observaties vinden plaats voor, tijdens en na een verzorging, worden uitgeschreven in een verslag en leiden tot individuele aanbevelingen die van belang zijn bij de verzorging van het individuele kind. Voorbeelden van mogelijke aanbevelingen zijn: het geven van time-outs tijdens een bepaald deel van de verzorging, het geven van de speen of iets om vast te houden, het betrekken van de ouders in de verzorging, het stimuleren van buidelen met de ouders (het kind ligt op de blote borst van een van de ouders) en het ondersteunen van de gebogen houding en bieden van veiligheid en grenzen door de handen over het lichaam van het kind te leggen (containen). Deze aanbevelingen worden besproken met de ouders en andere verzorgers van het kind. Daarbij worden ouders gestimuleerd om te kijken naar het individuele gedrag van het kind en actief betrokken te zijn bij de verzorging van hun kind.

NIDCAP onderzoeken in de Verenigde Staten en Zweden laten veelbelovende effecten zien. Echter, review artikelen over alle onderzoeken naar ontwikkelingsgerichte zorg geven aan dat er vaak gebruik gemaakt is van kleine onderzoeksgroepen en twijfelachtige methodiek. Zij adviseren grote gerandomiseerde onderzoeken in verschillende settings op te zetten om een volledig beeld van de effecten van ontwikkelingsgerichte zorg te krijgen. Door het arbeids- en kostenintensieve karakter van het NIDCAP, kiezen ziekenhuizen er soms voor om eerst alleen de basisaanbevelingen van ontwikkelingsgerichte zorg (vermindering van licht, geluid en activiteit en de ondersteuning van de ronde gebogen houding) toe te passen.

In dit proefschrift zijn de uitkomsten van twee opeenvolgende gerandomiseerde onderzoekstrials beschreven. De inclusieperiode liep van april 2000 tot augustus 2004, waarbij in de eerste fase 192 kinderen geïncludeerd werden en er in de tweede fase 168 kinderen geïncludeerd werden in een Nederlandse neonatale afdeling op twee locaties (het Leids Universitair Medisch Centrum (LUMC) in Leiden en het Juliana Kinderziekenhuis (JKZ) in Den Haag). In de eerste fase hebben wij gekeken naar de effecten van de basiselementen van ontwikkelingsgerichte zorg (het gebruik van gestandaardiseerde couveusehoezen en nestjes) in vergelijking met de standaard zorg op de afdeling. In de tweede fase hebben wij gekeken naar de effecten van de individuele NIDCAP interventie (met gedragsobservaties en individuele aanbevelingen) in vergelijking met de basiselementen van ontwikkelingsgerichte zorg. In dit proefschrift zijn de effecten van deze twee interventies op het gedrag en de gezondheidsgerelateerde kwaliteit van leven van het kind en de ervaringen van ouders en het personeel van de neonatologieafdeling beschreven.

Hoofdstuk 2 van dit proefschrift beschreef het effect van de basiselementen van ontwikkelingsgerichte zorg en de meer individuele NIDCAP interventie op de ouderlijke stress, het zelfvertrouwen en de door ouders ervaren steun van de verpleging tijdens de opname van het kind (ingevulde vragenlijsten, fase 1 =133, fase 2 =150). De NIDCAP interventie neigde het verschil in stress van moeder versus vader te verminderen, voornamelijk door een verhoging van de vaderlijke stress (p=.03). Dit zou wellicht verklaard kunnen worden door een verhoogde betrokkenheid van de vader in de zorg. Er werden geen effecten gevonden van beide interventies op ouderlijke stress, de door ouders ervaren steun van de verpleging en het zelfvertrouwen van moeder en vader.

Het effect van de basiselementen van ontwikkelingsgerichte zorg en de NIDCAP interventie op de gezondheidsgerelateerde kwaliteit van leven van het kind op 1 jarige leeftijd, gecorrigeerd voor de mate van vroeggeboorte, werd beschreven in **hoofdstuk 3**. De kinderen behaalden over het algemeen goed tot optimale gezondheidsgerelateerde kwaliteit van leven scores (ingevulde vragenlijsten fase 1 =136, fase 2 =128). Zowel de basiselementen van ontwikkelingsgerichte zorg als de NIDCAP interventie hadden geen effect op de door de ouders gerapporteerde gezondheidsgerelateerde kwaliteit van leven van de kinderen op 1 jarige leeftijd.

In **hoofdstuk 4** is gekeken naar het effect van de basiselementen van ontwikkelingsgerichte zorg, in vergelijking met de standaard zorg, op het gedrag van de kinderen en de ouderlijke stress op 1 en 2 jarige leeftijd, gecorrigeerd voor vroeggeboorte (ingevulde vragenlijsten 1 jaar =139, 2 jaar =133). Er werd een significant positief effect gevonden op het competentiegedrag en de vaardigheden van de kinderen op 1 jarige leeftijd (p=.009), voornamelijk met betrekking tot de motivatie om taken te beheersen (p=.002). Er werden geen significante effecten gevonden op probleemgedrag en ouderlijke stress op 1 en 2 jarige leeftijd. Er werd geconcludeerd dat de basiselementen van ontwikkelingsgerichte zorg een positief effect hebben op het competentiegedrag gedrag van te vroeg geboren kinderen op 1 jarige leeftijd.

Hoofdstuk 5 beschreef de effecten van de NIDCAP interventie met individuele gedragsobservaties en begeleiding, in vergelijking met de basiselementen van ontwikkelingsgerichte zorg, op het temperament op de gecorrigeerde leeftijd van 9 maanden (ingevulde vragenlijsten = 134) en het gedrag van het kind en de ouderlijke stress op 1 jarige leeftijd (ingevulde vragenlijsten = 128). Het NIDCAP lijkt het sociaal verwantschapsgedrag op 1 jaar te verbeteren (p=.011), vooral wanneer de duur van de opname op de afdelingen waar het onderzoek plaats vond langer was (interventieduur >1.5 maand, p=.006). Ouders gaven aan dat zij positieve effecten hadden ervaren van het NIDCAP op hun eigen ervaringen en het welzijn van hun kind tijdens de opname. Er werd echter geen significante verbetering van het temperament van het kind of de ouderlijke stress gevonden.

De evaluatie van de mening van het verpleegkundig en (para)medisch personeel over de implementatie van het NIDCAP, door middel van de twee onderzoekstrials op de neonatologie afdelingen in Leiden en Den Haag, werd beschreven in **hoofdstuk 6**. Het personeel (N=124) was over het algemeen positief over het NIDCAP en gaf aan verbeteringen te zien in het welzijn van de kinderen als een gevolg van de NIDCAP zorg. Het NIDCAP werd echter ook als tijdrovend gezien. Daarnaast zou NIDCAP een verslechtering van sommige werkomstandigheden kunnen veroorzaken. Het personeel gaf de noodzaak aan voor praktische begeleiding en continue informatievoorziening over relevante NIDCAP onderwerpen en onderzoek naar de effecten NIDCAP. Het verplegend personeel was significant positiever over het NIDCAP dan het medische personeel (p=.004). Deze bevindingen leidden tot de volgende aanbevelingen voor de implementatie van NIDCAP: toegankelijke informatievoorziening, continue klinische lessen en praktische begeleiding op de afdeling, een multi-disciplinair NIDCAP team en aanpak, discussie van de mogelijkheden ter verbetering van werkomstandigheden waar het NIDCAP een effect op kan hebben en een evaluatie van de tijdrovende aspecten van het NIDCAP.

In **hoofdstuk 7** werden tot slot de implicaties voor toekomstig onderzoek en de implementatie van het NIDCAP in Nederland bediscussieerd, naar aanleiding van de resultaten die in dit proefschrift beschreven zijn. Hoewel wij alleen kleine effecten vonden op de in dit proefschrift beschreven uitkomsten, geven de ouders en het verpleegkundig en (para)medisch personeel aan een positief effect te hebben ervaren op het comfort en welzijn van het kind tijdens opname. Een onderzoek in de Nederlandse setting naar het effect van een NIDCAP interventie met een langere interventieduur, en mogelijk ook thuisbezoeken, zou een interessant vervolg zijn op het huidige onderzoek. Andere uitkomsten (medisch en (neuro)ontwikkeling) van dit onderzoek die nog beschreven zullen worden en onderzoek in andere settings, zouden meer positieve effecten moeten aantonen. Een kostenbaten analyse zou moeten aantonen dat de positieve effecten zwaarder wegen dan de kosten van het NIDCAP. Tot dan is het aan te bevelen om alleen de minder intensieve basiselementen van ontwikkelingsgerichte zorg toe te passen zoals het gebruik van nestjes en couveusehoezen en het verminderen van het licht, geluid en de activiteit op de afdeling. Daarnaast kan het waardevol zijn om vanuit het NIDCAP observatieformulier en de synactieve theorie van ontwikkeling andere basisaanbevelingen te formuleren voor de verzorging van de kinderen en voor de training van het personeel.

Met bijzondere dank:

aan de kinderen en ouders
die zo enthousiast hebben meegedaan aan dit onderzoek,

het personeel van de neonatologieafdeling
in het Leids Universitair Medisch Centrum in Leiden
en het Juliana Kinderziekenhuis in Den Haag,

en aan alle mensen die hebben meegeholpen,
mijn familie

en István

zonder al jullie medewerking en steun
had dit proefschrift niet tot stand kunnen komen.

Curriculum Vitae

Sylvia Maria van der Pal werd op 27 april 1980 geboren te Leidschendam. In 1998 behaalde zij het eindexamen VWO aan het Alfrink College te Zoetermeer. Zij studeerde vervolgens van 1998 tot 2002 psychologie aan de Universiteit van Leiden. Aan deze universiteit werd in 2002 het doctoraal in de klinische en gezondheidspsychologie behaald.

Van 2002 tot 2003 werkte zij als data-assistent bij het Leids Ontwikkelingsgerichte Zorg Project in het Leids Universitair Medisch Centrum te Leiden. In april 2003 werd het promotietraject gestart bij het bovengenoemde onderzoek. In 2004 behaalde zij haar NIDCAP reliability examen. Van 2003 tot 2006 werd op de afdeling Neonatologie in het Leids Universitair Medisch Centrum aan dit proefschrift gewerkt. Per januari 2007 is zij werkzaam als junior onderzoeker bij TNO-Kwaliteit van Leven, Perinatologie en Voortplanting.

Printed in Dunstable, United Kingdom

91336857R00085